This book is useful for hi~~
reasons or
current m

D1262310

50 Ways
Women Can Prevent
Heart Disease

Other books by M. Sara Rosenthal:

50 Ways to Prevent Colon Cancer
The Thyroid Sourcebook
The Gynecological Sourcebook
The Pregnancy Sourcebook
The Fertility Sourcebook
The Breastfeeding Sourcebook
The Breast Sourcebook
The Gastrointestinal Sourcebook
Managing Your Diabetes
Managing Diabetes for Women
The Type 2 Diabetic Woman
The Thyroid Sourcebook for Women
Women & Depression

50 *Ways*
Women Can
Prevent Heart
Disease

M. Sara Rosenthal

Foreword by Laura Purdy, Ph.D.

LOWELL HOUSE

LOS ANGELES

NTC/Contemporary Publishing Group

The purpose of this book is to educate. It is sold with the understanding that the publisher and author shall have neither liability nor responsibility for any injury caused or alleged to be caused directly or indirectly by the information contained in this book. While every effort has been made to ensure its accuracy, the book's contents should not be construed as medical advice. Each person's health needs are unique. To obtain recommendations appropriate to your particular situation, please consult a qualified health care provider.

Library of Congress Cataloging-in-Publication Data
Rosenthal, M. Sara.
    50 ways women can prevent heart disease / M. Sara Rosenthal; foreword by Laura Purdy.
        p. cm.
    Includes bibliographical references and index.
    ISBN 0-7373-0502-9 (pbk.)
        1. Heart disease in women—Prevention. I. Title.

RC672.R6426 2000
616.1'205'082—dc21   00-056438

Published by Lowell House
A division of NTC/Contemporary Publishing Group, Inc.
4255 West Touhy Avenue, Lincolnwood, Illinois 60646-1975 U.S.A.

Printed in the United States of America

International Standard Book Number: 0-7373-0502-9

00 01 02 03 04 DHD 18 17 16 15 14 13 12 11 10 9 8 7 6 5 4 3 2 1

Contents

Foreword

When Sara Rosenthal asked me to write a foreword for this book, I felt both honored and excited. Honored, because it's not every day that people ask philosophers like me, who specialize in feminist medical ethics, to address women's heart disease in "the real world"! And excited, because her book will empower thousands of women to live longer, healthier lives.

In theory, this is a book that shouldn't have to exist. Our world could be organized to create conditions for good health naturally, by encouraging us to move our bodies, eat well, and not start smoking without our having to pay special attention. Medicine and health care could be geared to the needs of all humans, not focused—thirty years after the launch of *Ms.* magazine—on the 70-kilo white male. Research could take account of any differences between women and men, and therapies would be tested on women as well as men.

Because that world is still a dream, Sara Rosenthal provides you with the information you need to protect your body from heart disease by kicking bad habits (gooey desserts! smoking!) and taking up new ones (using both tried-and-true methods and new ones coming along the pike). Her book is full of tidbits that were new to me, even though I pride myself on being well informed about health maintenance. For instance, I learned why trans fats are bad, that yoga increases oxygen flow, that ibuprofen can increase blood pressure, and that high cholesterol has not been proven harmful to women.

But what's really special about this book is its attention to the broader social and political aspects of healthy living. It helps you understand how your environment makes it difficult to make good choices and provides suggestions about how to change the world so that others will find it easier to make wise ones. In particular, Sara Rosenthal is refreshingly up front about how sexism distorts the context of our decision making when it comes to matters of the heart. Read, enjoy, and learn!

—Laura Purdy, Ph.D., professor of medical ethics

Acknowledgments

I wish to thank the following people, whose expertise and dedication helped to lay so much of the groundwork for this book: Laura Purdy, Ph.D., has been writing about the ethics of varying standards of health care for women and men well before it was popular to comment on these matters. Looking at the ethical issues surrounding women's heart disease made many of the suggestions in this book possible, and I thank Dr. Purdy for repeating, in her foreword, what she has said in academic circles for years.

A number of past medical advisers on previous works helped me to shape the contents of this work. I wish to thank the following people (listed alphabetically): Gillian Arsenault, M.D., C.C.F.P., I.B.L.C., F.R.C.P.; Pamela Craig, M.D., F.A.C.S., Ph.D.; Masood Kahthamee, M.D., F.A.C.O.G.; Gary May, M.D., F.R.C.P.; James McSherry, M.B., Ch.B., F.C.F.P., F.R.C.G.P., F.A.A.F.P., F.A.B.M.P.; Suzanne Pratt, M.D., F.A.C.O.G.; and Robert Volpe, M.D., F.R.C.P., F.A.C.P.

William Harvey, Ph.D., L.L.B., University of Toronto Joint Centre for Bioethics, whose devotion to bioethics has inspired me, continues to support my work, and makes it possible for me to have the courage to question and challenge issues in health care and medical ethics. Irving Rootman, Ph.D., Director, University of Toronto Centre for Health Promotion, continues to encourage my interest in primary prevention and health promotion issues.

Larissa Kostoff, my editorial consultant, worked very hard to make this book a reality.

Introduction

The Signs of a Woman's Heart Attack

Heart disease is currently the number one cause of death in postmenopausal women; more women die of heart disease than of lung cancer or breast cancer. Half of all North Americans who die from heart attacks each year are women. But heart disease doesn't refer only to heart attacks; it includes strokes as well as a whole gamut of problems caused by poor circulation, known in clinical circles as *peripheral vascular disease,* or more plainly, "blood circulation disease." Peripheral vascular disease occurs when blood flow to the limbs (arms, legs, and feet) is blocked, which creates cramping, pains, or numbness. *In fact, pain and numbing in your arms or legs may be signs of heart disease or even an imminent heart attack.* A 1992 study reported that 20 percent of all women over age 60 suffered from peripheral vascular disease, and as more women approach menopause, that number will substantially increase.

One of the reasons for such high death rates from heart attacks among women is medical ignorance; most studies looking at heart disease have excluded women, which led to a myth that more men than women die of heart disease. The truth is more men die of heart attacks before age fifty, while more women die of heart attacks after age fifty, as a direct result of estrogen loss. Moreover, women who have had oopherectomies (removal of the ovaries) prior to natural menopause increase their risk of a heart attack *eightfold*. Since more women work outside the home than ever before, a number of experts cite stress as a major contributing factor to increased rates of heart disease in women.

Another problem is that women have different symptoms than men when it comes to heart disease, and so the "typical" warning signs we know about in men—angina, or chest pains—are often never present in women. In fact, chest pains in women are almost never related to heart disease. When symptoms of heart disease are not "male," many women are sent home to die—they are told that their heart attacks are "stress."

You're about to change all of that. Never before have so many women been at risk for heart disease. As millions of women turn fifty in 2000, the medical community will be forced to recognize the unique warning signs of heart disease and heart attacks in women. This book discusses all the *modifiable* risk factors for heart disease and the warning signs of a heart attack—in WOMEN. The major risk factors for women's heart disease are smoking, high blood pressure, obesity, and an inactive lifestyle. The Nurses' Health Study, a study that looked at 120,000 middle-aged women, found that women who were obese had two to three times more heart disease; this is particularly true for women with apple-shaped figures (meaning abdominal or upper body fat).

Studies show that hormone replacement therapy can help reduce your risk of heart disease. It is estrogen that protects women from heart disease prior to menopause; after menopause, the rates of heart disease in women soar as a result of estrogen loss. Lifestyle changes can significantly reduce your risk of heart disease, as well. Women who are physically active have a 60 to 75 percent lower risk of heart disease than inactive women. So modifying your lifestyle (by stopping smoking, eating less fat, and getting more exercise) can prevent heart and peripheral vascular disease. Blood pressure–lowering medications and, in select women, cholesterol-lowering drugs are other options.

In essence, this book is designed to help you prevent heart disease before it starts. But before I begin to show you the ways to prevent heart disease, the first thing you must know are warning signs to watch for. You see, for women, the symptoms of heart disease and even an actual heart attack can be vague—seemingly unrelated to heart problems. Signs of heart disease in women include some surprising symptoms:

- Shortness of breath and/or fatigue
- Jaw pain (often masked by arthritis and joint pain)
- Pain in the back of the neck (often masked by arthritis or joint pain)
- Pain down the right or left arm
- Back pain (often masked by arthritis and joint pain)
- Sweating (often masked by the discomforts of menopause)
- Fainting

- Palpitations
- Bloating (after menopause, would you believe this is a sign of coronary artery blockage?)
- Heartburn, belching, or other gastrointestinal pain (this is often a sign of an actual heart attack in women)
- Chest "heaviness" between the breasts; this is how women experience chest pain; some describe it as a sinking feeling or burning sensation, also described as an aching, throbbing, or a squeezing sensation, or a feeling that your heart jumps into your throat
- If you're diabetic, sudden swings in blood sugar
- Vomiting
- Confusion

If you now think you have heart disease, the following diagnostic tests can confirm it:

- Manual exam (doctor examining you with a stethoscope)
- Electrocardiogram
- Exercise stress test
- Echocardiogram
- Imaging tests that may use radioactive substances to take pictures of the heart

Now let's start counting the ways you can achieve a healthier heart and a higher quality of life.

Quitting Smoking

1. Know the Good Reasons to Quit Smoking

Roughly half a million North Americans die of smoking-related illnesses each year. That's 20 percent of *all* deaths from *all* causes. We already know that smoking causes lung cancer. But did you know that smokers are also *twice* as likely to develop heart disease? Consider other risk factors, such as estrogen loss, and you're at enormous danger of heart disease if you're a postmenopausal smoker. A single cigarette affects your body within seconds, increasing heart rate, blood pressure, and the demand for oxygen. The greater the demand for oxygen (because of constricted blood vessels and carbon monoxide, a by-product of cigarettes), the greater the risk of heart disease.

Lesser-known long-term effects of smoking include lowering of HDL, or "good" cholesterol, and damage to the lining of blood vessel walls, which pave the way for arterial plaque formation. In addition to increasing your risk for lung cancer and heart disease, smoking can lead to stroke, peripheral vascular disease, and a host of other cancers.

Take a look at some of the things you'll gain by quitting smoking:

- Decreased risk of heart disease

- Decreased risk of cancer (that includes lung, esophagus, mouth, throat, pancreas, kidney, bladder, and cervix)
- Lower heart rate and blood pressure
- Decreased risk of lung disease (bronchitis, emphysema)
- Relaxation of blood vessels
- Improved sense of smell and taste
- Better teeth
- Fewer wrinkles

2. Understand "Smoke and Mirrors": The Connection Between Weight and Smoking

Smoking and obesity often coexist. Women frequently begin to smoke in their teens as a way to lose weight. A 1997 study done by the Department of Psychology and Preventive Medicine at the University of Memphis in Tennessee shows that this approach doesn't work. Smoking teens are just as likely to become obese over time as non-smokers. Ironically, it was found that the more a person weighed, the more cigarettes he or she smoked. Many women use nicotine as a "weight loss" drug. They will either use it for initial weight loss, or worse, revisit the habit long after they've quit to achieve the same goal.

Smoking satisfies "mouth hunger"—the need to have something in your mouth. It also causes withdrawal symptoms that can drive people to eat. If you need to lose weight, also smoke, and have just one additional risk factor for heart disease, such as high blood pressure or high blood sugar, something has got to give! Smoking will restrict small blood vessels, which can put you at much greater risk for heart disease. There are, unfortunately, no easy answers to the dilemma of weight loss versus quitting smoking. Most health care providers will assess your current risk of heart disease and/or stroke and help you prioritize your lifestyle changes. Looking into a credible smoking cessation program is one answer. But most women will only quit smoking when faced with the reality of a terminal illness. In other words, fear is often the best motivator.

3. Know How Your Smoking Can Hurt Your Family

Most women don't like to be told this bit of news, but it's often what they need to hear to quit smoking once and for all. As women, we are born nurturers, and when we see that our behavior is hurting someone else, often this is motivation enough to modify it. So brace yourself—your second-hand smoke, also known as passive smoking, or more recently, environmental tobacco smoke (ETS), can cause serious illness and cancers in the people you love the most: your children, partners, and spouses. What most smokers don't understand about tobacco and smoking is that non-smokers are vulnerable to tobacco-related illnesses as well. Secondhand smoke is recognized as a leading cause of lung cancer in nonsmokers and respiratory problems in young children and adults. Did you know, for example, that hundreds of North Americans die each year from lung cancer caused by environmental tobacco smoke?

The 1986 report of the U.S. surgeon general concluded that involuntary exposure to secondhand smoke could cause tobacco-related diseases, including lung cancer. This landmark document proved that no one is without risk. It was this document that changed the focus of abstaining from smoking from a lifestyle issue to an environmental health hazard.

A recent report from the U.S. Environmental Protection Agency (EPA) has confirmed the surgeon general's conclusions by classifying ETS as a Class A carcinogen, the most deadly category of cancer-causing agents. The report found that ETS, which is a combination of sidestream and exhaled smoke, causes lung cancer in nonsmokers and impairs the health of infants and children.

Pregnancy and Infants

Fetuses and children whose parents smoke are the most vulnerable to ETS. Respiratory illnesses are more common in children born to smokers than those of nonsmokers, while smoking during pregnancy can lead to the premature rupture of membranes, premature birth, perinatal death, placental abnormalities, and bleeding during pregnancy.

Breastfeeding mothers who smoke will find their milk supply affected by nicotine. Consequently, they may need to stop breastfeeding, thus depriving their children of the benefits of breastfeeding and exposing them to the dangers of formula feeding. The American Academy of Pediatrics lists any amount of nicotine as "contraindicated" (harmful) during breastfeeding. Too much nicotine can cause shock, vomiting, diarrhea, rapid heart rate, and restlessness in the baby. Secondhand smoke is perhaps even *more* damaging to your baby than high nicotine levels in breast milk. There are oodles of studies that conclude, "Yes, babies who breathe in smoke from one or both parents don't feel as well as babies born to nonsmokers." Secondhand smoke can cause pneumonia, bronchitis, or even SIDS (Sudden Infant Death Syndrome).

4. Look into a Variety of Smoking Cessation Programs

Not everyone can quit smoking cold turkey, although it's a strategy that many have used successfully. (Some cold turkey quitters report that keeping one package of cigarettes within reach lessens anxiety.) The symptoms of nicotine withdrawal begin within a few hours and peak twenty-four to forty-eight hours after quitting. You may experience anxiety, irritability, hostility, restlessness, insomnia, and anger. For these reasons, many smokers turn to smoking cessation programs, which can include some of the following:

- *Behavioral counseling:* Behavioral counseling, either group or individual, can raise the abstinence rate to 20 to 25 percent. This approach to smoking cessation aims to change the mental processes of the smoker, reinforce the benefits of nonsmoking, and teach skills to help the smoker resist the urge to smoke.

- *Nicotine gum:* Nicotine (Nicorette) gum is now available over the counter. It works as an aid to help you quit smoking by reducing nicotine cravings and withdrawal symptoms. Nicotine gum helps you wean yourself from nicotine by allowing you to gradually decrease the dosage until you stop using it altogether, a process that usually takes about twelve weeks. The only disadvantage of this method is that it continues the oral and addictive aspects of smoking (rewarding the urge to smoke with a dose of nicotine).

- *Nicotine patch:* Transdermal nicotine, or the "patch" (Habitrol, Nicoderm, Nicotrol) doubles abstinence rates for former smokers. Most brands are now available over the counter. Each morning, a new patch is applied to a different area of dry, clean, hairless skin and left on for the day. Some patches are designed to be worn a full twenty-four hours. The constant supply of nicotine to the bloodstream, however, sometimes causes very vivid or disturbing dreams. You can also expect to feel a mild itching, burning, or tingling at the site of the patch when it is first applied. The nicotine patch works best when it is worn for at least seven to twelve weeks, with a gradual decrease in strength (less nicotine). Many smokers find it effective because it allows them to tackle the psychological addiction to smoking before they are forced to deal with physical symptoms of withdrawal.

- *Nicotine inhaler:* The nicotine inhaler (Nicotrol Inhaler) delivers nicotine orally via inhalation from a plastic tube. Its success rate is about 28 percent, similar to that of nicotine gum. It's available by prescription only in the United States and has yet to make its debut in Canada. Like nicotine gum, the inhaler mimics smoking behavior by responding to each craving or urge to smoke, a feature that has both advantages and disadvantages for the smoker who wants to get over the physical symptoms of withdrawal. The nicotine inhaler should be used for a period of twelve weeks.

- *Nicotine nasal spray:* Like nicotine gum and the nicotine patch, the nasal spray reduces craving and withdrawal symptoms, allowing smokers to cut back gradually. One squirt delivers about 1 mg nicotine. In three clinical trials involving 730 patients, 31 to 35 percent were not smoking after six months. This compares to an average of 12 to 15 percent of smokers who were able to quit unaided. The nasal spray has a couple of advantages over the gum and the patch: Nicotine is rapidly absorbed across the nasal membranes, providing a kick that is more like the "real thing"; and the prompt onset of action plus a flexible dosing schedule benefits heavier smokers. Because the nicotine reaches the bloodstream so quickly, nasal sprays do have a greater potential for addiction than the slower-acting gum and patch. Nasal sprays are not yet available for use in Canada.

- *Alternative therapies:* Hypnosis, meditation, and acupuncture have helped some smokers quit. In the case of hypnosis and meditation, sessions may be private or part of a group smoking cessation program.

5. Ask About Drugs That May Aid in Smoking Cessation

The drug bupropion hydrochloride (Zyban) is now available and is an option for people who have been unsuccessful using nicotine replacement. Formerly prescribed as an antidepressant, bupropion was discovered by accident; researchers knew that smokers trying to quit were often depressed, so they began experimenting with the drug as a means to fight depression, not addiction. Bupropion reduces the withdrawal symptoms associated with smoking cessation and can be used in conjunction with nicotine replacement therapy. Researchers suspect that bupropion works directly in the brain to disrupt the addictive power of nicotine by affecting the same chemical neurotransmitters (or messengers) in the brain, such as dopamine, that nicotine does.

The pleasurable effects of addictive drugs such as nicotine and cocaine result from the release of dopamine.
Smoking floods the brain with dopamine. The *New England
Journal of Medicine* published the results of a study of more
than six hundred smokers taking bupropion. At the end of
treatment, 44 percent of those who took the highest dose of
the drug (300 mg) were not smoking, compared to 19 percent of the group who took a placebo. By the end of one
year, 23 percent of the 300 mg group and 12 percent of the
placebo group were still smoke free. Using Zyban *with* nicotine replacement therapy seems to improve the quit rate a
bit further. Four-week quit rates from the study were 23
percent for the placebo; 36 percent for the patch; 49 percent
for Zyban; and 58 percent for the combination of Zyban
and the patch.

6. Win the War on Tobacco

Don't let the tobacco companies win! Get mad, and take
back your life. When smokers hear the following facts,
many of them get so angry, they quit. So I tell you these
things not to punish you, but to motivate you. It's been long
known that unethical practices occur in the tobacco industry, such as:

- Suppressing evidence linking tobacco with ill health.
- Using nicotine to enhance the addictive properties of
  tobacco. Cigarette manufacturing, in this case,
  becomes all about "nicotine delivery."
- Circulating misleading information masking the
  health consequences of smoking.
- Using advertising that targets vulnerable groups.
  These ad campaigns sink to terrible lows in order to

appeal to children, young women, and low-income individuals.

- Exporting tobacco products to Third World nations, often with accompanying advertising aimed at minors or other groups who don't have the income to support a nicotine addiction.

7. Use Your Feminism to Help You Quit Smoking

As a woman, it's important to realize that tobacco companies use young women's body image dilemmas as tools to addict them early to nicotine, which has devastating health consequences for you, as a smoker, and for your daughter, who may well be smoking when you're not looking. The results of numerous studies show that most young women begin smoking to *control their weight*. (See number 2). Ninety percent of all eating disorders are diagnosed in women. A *New York Times* poll found that 36 percent of girls aged thirteen to seventeen wanted to change their looks. A 1995 survey of girls in grades nine through twelve conducted by the Centers for Disease Control found that 60 percent of them were trying to lose weight and that 5 to 10 percent of girls aged fourteen and over suffer from eating disorders.

Tobacco ads in women's magazines continue to sell the message to young women that smoking is "beautiful" or "glamorous." One brand, as of 1999, sported the copy "It's a woman's thing," showing a beautiful, thin woman in a natural setting. Boycotting women's magazines that accept tobacco ads is one thing you, as a consumer, can do to stop this trend; writing the magazine's publisher and editor, explaining why you're boycotting their publication, will do a lot to end this practice. Tobacco companies have also sponsored fashion and other women-related events. Boycotting these events and sending letters to the organizations explaining your reasons for your actions are important acts of protest you, as a consumer—and a woman, have the power to carry out.

Most important, quitting smoking, and recognizing all the social pressures that helped addict you, is a way to counteract the existence of smoking as a sort of marketing violence against women that ought not be allowed to continue. Talk to your daughters and nieces and granddaughters about this form of marketing abuse, and try to end the cycle and prevent their addiction.

8. Quit Cigar Smoking, Too

Cigar smoking is in vogue for those in the "know," in the "money," or those who want to be "cool." It is a dangerous trend that is capturing the interest of millions of privileged women. When you smoke a cigar, you're getting filler, binder, and wrapper, which are made of air-cured and fermented tobaccos. Like cigarette tobacco, lit cigars emit over four thousand chemicals, of which forty-three are known to cause cancer.

Cigar smokers have higher death rates than nonsmokers for most smoking-related diseases, although not nearly as high as those of cigarette smokers. When the nicotine is absorbed through the mouth, however, cigar/pipe smokers, as well as anyone using chewing tobacco or snuff, are at higher risk of laryngeal, oral, and esophageal cancer. Cigar/pipe smokers also have higher death rates than nonsmokers from chronic obstructive lung disease as well as lung cancer.

Cigar smoking is a pastime that is being sold to women as something that is attractive and sexy. And women are actually buying into it, when in fact they are much more attracted to the maleness of the cigar and the male world it seems to evoke for them. A cigar is *not* just a cigar!

9. Try to Get Reimbursed for Your Quitting Costs

Since tobacco companies have so much money to "burn," how about focusing on *good* ways to spend it? North Americans spend billions of dollars per year to treat people with smoking-related illnesses, such as heart disease and lung cancer. This is an enormous economic burden placed on society, especially when you consider the fact that *prevention is possible.* Did you know that you may be able to recover your costs for quitting and be compensated for harms? Several states in the United States have now launched lawsuits against the tobacco industry. In 1998, following the publication of the *Vanity Fair* article "The Man Who Knew Too Much," lawsuits against "big tobacco" were filed first by Mississippi, then by forty other states; they were eventually settled at $246 billion. Anyone attempting to quit smoking through the smoking cessation methods delineated in number 4 should request reimbursement from her cigarette brand manufacturer. You should also seek out other quitters who may want to launch a class-action suit to recover smoking cessation costs from tobacco manufacturers. You may also want to ask your employer to fund a smoking cessation program, seeking financial support from tobacco companies (or using tobacco money the government accumulates to fund the smoking cessation program).

10. Realize the Personal and Political Gains of Quitting

Quitting smoking is the most important step you can take to lower your risk of heart disease. So the earlier you quit, the sooner you can start to see the results. That said, it's important not to expect miracles; studies show that any real health benefits long-term ex-smokers gain from quitting (that is, people who smoked from their teen years until age fifty-five or so) were not noticeable until at least fifteen years after they quit. The American Cancer Society's Cancer Prevention Study noted that the death rates of former smokers did not begin to match those of never-smokers until fifteen to twenty years after the smokers quit. If you smoked for only a short period of time, or quit smoking in your thirties or forties, the health benefits will be realized much more quickly. So the sooner you quit, the better!

Your quitting is also an important way to prevent future generations from getting hooked. To eliminate smoking-related lung cancer (which accounts for 70 percent of lung cancers) and other smoking-related diseases, we have to focus on preventing people from starting. Your quitting contributes momentum to antismoking campaigns and messages, and it also helps to save a little bit of the world. Smoke that doesn't blow from your mouth into the air contributes to a decrease in a significant source of environmental pollution.

Diet

11. Understand Fat

Fat is technically known as *fatty acids*, which are crucial nutrients for our cells. We cannot live without fatty acids, or fat. If you looked at each fat molecule carefully, you'd find three different kinds of fatty acids on it: saturated (solid), monounsaturated (less solid, with the exception of olive and peanut oils), and polyunsaturated (liquid) fatty acids. When you see the term *unsaturated fat,* this refers to either monounsaturated or polyunsaturated fats.

These three fatty acids combine with glycerol to make what are chemically known as triglycerides. Each fat molecule is a link chain made up of glycerol, carbon atoms, and hydrogen atoms. The more hydrogen atoms on that chain, the more saturated or solid the fat. The liver breaks down fat molecules by secreting bile (stored in the gall-bladder—its sole function). The liver also makes cholesterol. Too much saturated fat may cause your liver to overproduce cholesterol, while the triglycerides in your bloodstream will rise, perpetuating the problem.

Fat is a good thing—in moderation. But like all good things, most of us want too much of it. Excess dietary fat is by far the most damaging element in the Western diet. A gram of fat contains twice the calories as the same amount of protein or carbohydrate. Decreasing the fat in your diet and replacing it with more grain products, vegetables, and fruit is the best way to lower your risk of colon cancer and cardiovascular diseases. Fat in the diet comes from meats, dairy products, and vegetable oils. Other sources of fat include coconuts (60 percent fat), peanuts (78 percent fat), and avocados (82 percent fat). There are different kinds of fatty acids in these sources of fats: saturated, monounsaturated, and polyunsaturated, as described above. There is also a fourth kind of fat in our diets: trans-fatty acids. These are factory-made fats found in margarines, for example (discussed in number 12).

To cut through all this big, fat jargon, you can boil down fat into two categories: harmful fats and helpful fats (the popular press often defines these as "good fats/bad fats").

Harmful Fats

The following are harmful fats because they can increase your risk of cardiovascular problems, as well as many cancers, including colon and breast cancers. These are fats that are fine in moderation but harmful in excess (and harmless if not eaten at all):

- *Saturated fats.* These are solid at room temperature and stimulate cholesterol production in your body. In fact, the way that saturated fat looks prior to ingesting it is the way it will look when it lines your arteries. Foods high in saturated fat include processed meat, fatty meat, lard, butter, margarine, solid vegetable shortening, chocolate, and tropical oils (coconut oil is more than 90 percent saturated). Saturated fat should be consumed only in very small amounts.

- *Trans-fatty acids.* These are factory-made fats that behave just like saturated fat in your body. See number 22 for details.

Helpful Fats

These are fats that are beneficial to your health, and actually protect against certain illnesses, such as cardiovascular disease. You are encouraged to use these fats more, rather than less, frequently in your diet. In fact, nutritionists suggest that you substitute these for harmful fats.

- *Unsaturated fat.* This is partially solid or liquid at room temperature. The more liquid the fat, the more polyunsaturated it is, which, in fact, *lowers* your cholesterol levels. This group of fats includes monounsaturated fats and polyunsaturated fats. Sources of unsaturated fats include vegetable oils (canola, safflower, sunflower, corn) and seeds and nuts. Unsaturated fats come from all plants (with the exception of tropical oils, such as coconut—these are saturated).

- *Fish fats (omega-3 oils).* The fats naturally present in fish that swim in cold waters, known as omega-3 fatty acids or fish oils, are all polyunsaturated. Again, polyunsaturated fats are good for you; they lower cholesterol levels, are crucial for brain tissue, and protect against heart disease. Look for cold-water fish such as mackerel, albacore tuna, salmon, and sardines.

12. Avoid Factory-Made Fats

An assortment of factory-made fats have been introduced into our diet, courtesy of food producers who are trying to give us the taste of fat without all the calories of saturated fats. Unfortunately, man-made fats offer their own bag of horrors. That's because when a fat is made in a factory, it becomes a trans-fatty acid, a harmful fat that *not only* raises the level of "bad" cholesterol (LDL, short for low-density lipoprotein) in your bloodstream, but lowers the amount of "good" cholesterol (HDL, short for high-density lipoprotein) that's already there.

How, exactly, does a trans-fatty acid come into being? Trans-fatty acids are what you get when you make a liquid oil, such as corn oil, into a more solid or spreadable substance, such as margarine. Trans-fatty acids, you might say, are the "road to hell, paved with good intentions." Someone, way back when, thought that if you could take the good fat—unsaturated fat—and solidify it, so it could double as butter or lard, you could eat the same things without missing the spreadable fat. That sounds like a great idea. Unfortunately, to make an unsaturated liquid fat more solid, you have to add hydrogen to its molecules. This is known as *hydrogenation*, the process that converts liquid fat to semisolid fat. Hydrogenated palm oil, that ever-popular chocolate bar ingredient, is a classic example of a trans-fatty acid. Hydrogenation also prolongs the shelf life of fats, such as polyunsaturated fats, which can oxidize when exposed to air, causing rancid odors or flavors. Deep-frying oils used in the restaurant trade are generally hydrogenated.

What's Wrong with Trans-fatty Acid?

Trans-fatty acid is sold as a polyunsaturated or monounsaturated fat with a line of advertising copy such as, "Made from polyunsaturated vegetable oil." The problem is, in your body, it is treated as a *saturated* fat. So really, trans-fatty acids are a saturated fat in disguise. The advertiser may, in fact, say that the product contains "no saturated fat" or is "healthier" than the comparable animal or tropical oil product with saturated fat. So be careful out there: *Read your labels.* The magic word you're looking for is "hydrogenated." If the product lists a variety of unsaturated fats (monounsaturated X oil, polyunsaturated Y oil, and so on), keep reading. If the word *hydrogenated* appears, count that product as a saturated fat; your body will!

Margarine versus Butter

There's an old tongue twister: "Betty Botter bought some butter that made the batter bitter; so Betty Botter bought more butter that made the batter better." Are we making our batters bitter or better with margarine? It depends.

Since the news of trans-fatty acids broke in the late 1980s, margarine manufacturers began to offer some less "bitter" margarines; some contain no hydrogenated oils, while others have much smaller amounts. Margarines with less than 60 to 80 percent oil (9 to 11 grams of fat) will contain 1.0 to 3.0 grams of trans-fatty acids per serving, compared to butter, which is 53 percent saturated fat. You might say it's merely a choice between a bad fat and a *worse* fat.

It's also possible for a liquid vegetable oil to retain a high concentration of unsaturated fat when it's been partially hydrogenated. In this case, your body will metabolize it as some saturated fat and some unsaturated fat.

Fake Fat

We have artificial sweeteners; why not artificial fat? This question has led to the creation of an emerging yet highly suspicious ingredient: the *fat substitute,* designed to replace real fat and hence reduce the calories from real fat without compromising the taste. This is done by creating a fake fat that the body cannot absorb.

One of the first fat substitutes was Simplesse, an all-natural fat substitute, made from milk and egg-white protein, which was developed by the NutraSweet Company. Simplesse apparently adds 1 to 2 calories per gram instead of the usual 9 calories per gram from fat. Other fat substitutes simply take protein and carbohydrates and modify them in some way to simulate the textures of fat (creamy, smooth, and so on). All these fat substitutes help to create low-fat products.

The calorie-free fat substitute now being promoted is called olestra, developed by Procter and Gamble. It's currently being test marketed in the United States in a variety of savory snacks such as potato chips and crackers. Olestra is a potentially dangerous ingredient that most experts feel can do more harm than good. Canada has not yet approved it.

Olestra is made from a combination of vegetable oils and sugar. It tastes just like the real thing, but the biochemical structure is a molecule too big for your liver to break down. So, olestra just gets passed into the large intestine and is excreted. Olestra is more than an "empty" molecule, however. According to the FDA Commissioner of Food and

Drugs, olestra may cause diarrhea and cramps and may deplete your body of vital nutrients, including vitamins A, D, E, and K, necessary for blood clotting. Indeed, all studies conducted by Procter & Gamble have shown this potential. If the FDA approves olestra for use as a cooking-oil substitute, you'll see it in every imaginable high-fat product. There is another danger with olestra, however, which nutritionists raised in a critique of olestra published in a 1996 issue of the *University of California at Berkley Wellness Letter* (the year olestra was approved for test markets). Instead of encouraging people to choose nutritious foods, such as fruits, grains, and vegetables, over high-fat foods, products like these encourage a high fake-fat diet that's still too low in fiber and other essential nutrients. The no-fat icing on the cake is that these people could potentially wind up with a vitamin deficiency to boot. Products such as olestra should make you nervous.

13. Cut Down on Carbohydrates

Fat is not the only thing that can make you fat. *What about carbohydrates?* You see, a diet high in carbohydrates can also make you fat. That's because carbohydrates—meaning starchy stuff, such as rice, pasta, breads, and potatoes—can be stored as fat when eaten in excess.

Carbohydrates can be simple or complex. Simple carbohydrates are found in any food that has natural sugar (honey, fruits, juices, vegetables, milk) and anything that contains table sugar.

Complex carbohydrates are more sophisticated foods that are made up of larger molecules, such as grain foods, starches, and foods high in fiber.

Normally, all carbs convert to glucose when you eat them. Glucose is the technical term for simplest sugar. All your energy comes from glucose in your blood—also known as blood glucose or blood sugar—your body fuel. When your blood sugar is used up, you feel weak and tired . . . and hungry. What happens, though, when you eat more carbohydrates than your body can use? Your body will store those extra carbs as fat. What we also know is that the rate at which glucose is absorbed by your body from carbohydrates is affected by other components of your meal, such as protein, fiber, and fat. If you're eating only carbohydrates and no protein or fat, for example, they will convert into glucose more quickly, to the point where you may feel mood swings, as your blood sugar rises and dips.

Nutrition experts advise that you should consume roughly 50 to 55 percent carbohydrates, 15 to 20 percent protein, and less than 30 percent fat daily of your total intake for a healthy diet.

14. Understand Sugar

Sugars are found naturally in many of the foods you eat. As mentioned above, the simplest form of sugar is called glucose. You can buy pure glucose at any drugstore in the form of dextrose tablets. Dextrose is just "edible glucose." For example, when you see people having sugar water fed to them intravenously, dextrose is the sugar in that water. When you see dextrose on a candy-bar label, it means that the candy-bar manufacturer used edible glucose in the recipe.

Glucose is the baseline ingredient of all naturally occurring sugars, which include:

- *Sucrose:* table or white sugar, naturally found in sugar cane and sugar beets
- *Fructose:* the natural sugar in fruits and vegetables
- *Lactose:* the natural sugar in all milk products
- *Maltose:* the natural sugar in grains (flours and cereals)

When you ingest a natural sugar of any kind, you're actually ingesting one part glucose and one or two parts of *another* naturally occurring sugar. For example, sucrose is biochemically constructed from one part glucose and one part fructose. So, from glucose it came, and unto glucose it shall return—once it hits your digestive system. The same is true for all naturally occurring sugars, with the exception of lactose. As it happens, lactose breaks down into glucose and an "odd duck" simple sugar, galactose (which I used to think was something in our solar system until I became a health writer). Just think of lactose as the Milky Way, and you'll probably remember.

Simple sugars can get pretty complicated when you discuss their molecular structures. For example, simple sugars can be classified as monosaccharides (single sugars) or dissaccharides (double sugars). But unless you're writing a chemistry exam on sugars, you don't need to know this confusing stuff; you just need to know that all naturally occurring sugars wind up as glucose once you eat them. Glucose is carried to your cells through the bloodstream and is used as body fuel or energy.

How long does it take for one of the above sugars to return to glucose? It greatly depends on the amount of fiber in your food, how much protein you've eaten, and how much fat accompanies the sugar in your meal. As stated in number 23, if you have enough energy or fuel, once that sugar becomes glucose, it can be stored as fat. And that's how—and why—sugar can make you fat.

Factory-Added Sugars

What you have to watch out for is *added sugar;* these are sugars that manufacturers add to foods during processing or packaging. Foods containing fruit juice concentrates, invert sugar, regular corn syrup, honey or molasses, hydrolyzed lactose syrup, or high-fructose corn syrup (made from highly concentrated fructose through the hydrolysis of starch) all have added sugars. Many people don't realize, however, that pure, *unsweetened* fruit juice is still a potent source of sugar, even when it contains no added processed sugar. Extra lactose (naturally occurring sugar in milk products), dextrose (edible glucose), and maltose (naturally occurring sugar in grains) are also contained in many of your foods. In other words, the products may have naturally occurring sugars anyway, and then *more* sugar is thrown in to enhance consistency, taste, and so on. The best way to know how much sugar is in a product is to look at the nutritional label for "carbohydrates."

Sweeteners

Here's what you need to know about sweeteners if you're trying to cut down on fat. While artificial sweeteners do not contain sugar (for diabetics, this means they will not affect blood sugar levels), they *may* contain a tiny amount of calories. It depends on whether that sweetener is classified as nutritive or nonnutritive.

Nutritive sweeteners have calories or contain natural sugar. White or brown table sugar, molasses, honey, and syrup are all considered nutritive sweeteners. *Sugar alcohols* are also nutritive sweeteners because they are made from fruits or produced commercially from dextrose. Sorbitol, mannitol, xylitol, and maltitol are all sugar alcohols. Sugar alcohols contain only 4 calories per gram, like ordinary sugar, and will affect your blood sugar levels like ordinary sugar. Their effects depend on how much is consumed and the degree of absorption from your digestive tract.

Nonnutritive sweeteners are sugar substitutes or artificial sweeteners; they do not have any calories and will not affect your blood sugar levels. Examples of nonnutritive sweeteners are saccharin, cyclamate, aspartame, sucralose, and acesulfame potassium.

Aspartame was invented in the 1980s, and is sold as NutraSweet. It was considered a nutritive sweetener because it was derived from natural sources (two amino acids, aspartic acid and phenylalanine), which means that aspartame is digested and metabolized the same way as any other protein food. For every gram of aspartame, there are 4 calories. But since aspartame is two hundred times sweeter than sugar, you don't need very much of it to achieve the desired sweetness. In at least ninety countries, aspartame is found in more than 150 product categories, including breakfast cereals, beverages, desserts, candy and gum, syrups, salad dressings, and various snack foods. Here's where it gets confusing: Aspartame is also available as a tabletop sweetener under the brand names Equal and, most recently, PROSWEET. An interesting point about aspartame is that it's not recommended for baking or any other recipe where heat is required. The two amino acids in it separate with heat and the product loses its sweetness. It's not harmful if heated, but your recipe won't turn out right.

For the moment, aspartame is considered safe for everybody, including people with diabetes, pregnant women, and children. The only people who are cautioned against consuming it are those with a rare hereditary disease known as phenylketonuria (PKU) because aspartame contains phenylalanine, which people with PKU cannot tolerate.

Another common tabletop sweetener is sucralose, sold as Splenda. Splenda is a white crystalline powder, actually made from sugar itself. It's six hundred times sweeter than table sugar but is not broken down in your digestive system, so it has no calories at all. Splenda can also be used in hot or cold foods and is found in hot and cold beverages, frozen foods, baked goods, and other packaged foods.

In the United States, you can still purchase cyclamate, a nonnutritive sweetener sold under the brand name Sucaryl or Sugar Twin. Cyclamate is also the sweetener used in many weight control products; it is thirty times sweeter than table sugar, with no aftertaste. Cyclamate is fine for hot or cold foods. In Canada, however, you can only find cyclamate as Sugar Twin or as a sugar substitute used in medications.

Sugar Alcohols

Not to be confused with alcoholic beverages, sugar alcohols are nutritive sweeteners, like regular sugar. These are found naturally in fruits or manufactured from carbohydrates. Sorbitol, mannitol, xylitol, maltitol, maltitol syrup, lactitol, isomalt, and hydrogenated starch hydrolysates are all sugar alcohols. In your body, these types of sugars are absorbed lower down in the digestive tract and will cause gastrointestinal symptoms if you use too much. Because sugar alcohols are absorbed more slowly, they were once touted as ideal for people with diabetes, but since they are carbohydrates, they still increase your blood sugar level, just like regular sugar. Now that artificial sweeteners are on the market in abundance, the only real advantage of sugar alcohols is that they don't cause cavities. The bacteria in your mouth doesn't like sugar alcohols as much as real sugar.

According to the FDA, even foods that contain sugar alcohols can be labeled "sugar free." Sugar alcohol products can also be labeled "does not promote tooth decay," which is often confused with "low calorie."

15. Learn to Interpret Food Labels

Since 1993, food labels must adhere to strict guidelines set out by the Food and Drug Administration (FDA) and the U.S. Department of Agriculture's (USDA) Food Safety and Inspection Service (FSIS). All labels list "Nutrition Facts" on the side or back of the package. The "% Daily Values" column tells you how high or low that food is in various nutrients, such as fat, saturated fat, and cholesterol. A number of 5 or less is low; good news if the product shows <5 for fat, saturated fat, and cholesterol, bad news if the product is <5 for fiber. Serving sizes are also confusing. Foods that are similar are given the same *type* of serving size defined by the FDA. That means that five cereals that all weigh X grams per cup will share the same serving sizes.

Calories (how much energy) and calories from fat (how much fat) are also listed per serving of food. Total carbohydrate, dietary fiber, sugars, other carbohydrates (which means starches), total fat, saturated fat, cholesterol, sodium, potassium, and vitamins and minerals are given in Percent Daily Values, based on the 2,000-calorie diet recommended by the U.S. government. (In Canada, Recommended

Nutrient Intake [RNI] is used for vitamins and minerals, while ingredients on labels are listed according to weight, with the "most" listed first.)

That's not where the confusion ends—*or even begins!* You have to wade through the various claims on the label and understand what they mean. For example, anything that is "X free" (as in sugar free, saturated fat free, cholesterol free, sodium free, calorie free, and so on) means that the product indeed has no X or that X is so tiny, it is insignificant. This is not the same thing as a label that says "95 percent fat free." In this case, the product contains relatively small amounts of fat, but still has fat. This claim is based on 100 grams of the product. For example, if a snack food contains 2.5 grams of fat per 50 grams, it can be said to be "95 percent fat free."

A label that screams "low in saturated fat" or "low in calories" is *not* fat free or calorie free. It means that you can eat a large amount of that food without exceeding the Daily Value for that food. In potato-chip country, that could mean you can eat twelve potato chips instead of six. So if you eat the whole bag of low-fat chips, you're still eating a lot of fat. Be sure to check serving sizes.

"Cholesterol free" or "low cholesterol" means that the product doesn't have any, or much, animal fat (hence, cholesterol). This doesn't mean "low fat." Pure vegetable oil doesn't come from animals but is pure fat!

Less and More

Then there are the comparison claims, such as "fewer," "reduced," "less," "more," or, my favorite, "light" (or worse, "lite"!). These words appear on foods that have been nutritionally altered from a previous version or a competitor's version. For example, Brand X Potato Chips—Regular may have much more fat than Brand X Potato Chips—Lite "with less fat than regular Brand X." That doesn't mean that Brand X Lite is fat free, or even low in fat. It just means it's B percent *lower* in fat than Brand X Regular.

On the flip side, Brand Y may have a trace amount of calcium, while Brand Y—"now with more calcium" may still have a small amount of calcium, but 10 percent more than Brand Y. (In other words, you may still need to eat a hundred bowls of Brand Y before you get the daily requirement for calcium!)

To be light or "lite" a product has to contain either one-third fewer calories or half the fat of the regular product. Or, a low-calorie or low-fat food contains 50 percent less sodium. Something that is "light in sodium" means it has at least 50 percent less sodium than the regular product, such as canned soup. (But if you're buying hair color that reads "light brown," it is a descriptive word, not referring to an ingredient!)

Planning to pick up some cough syrup for that cold of yours when you hit the pharmacy section? How about vitamin pills? Check the sugar content first. Your pharmacist can recommend a sugar-free remedy.

Sugar Free

When a label says "sugar free," the food contains less than 0.5 grams of sugars per serving, while a "reduced-sugar" food contains at least 25 percent less sugar per serving than the regular product. If the label also states that the product is not a reduced- or low-calorie food, or it is not for weight control, it's got enough sugar in there to make you think twice.

But sugar free in the language of labels simply means "sucrose free." That doesn't mean the product is *carbohydrate free*, as in dextrose free, lactose free, glucose free, or fructose free. Check the labels for all things ending in "ose" to find out the sugar content; you're not just looking for sucrose. Watch out for "no added sugar," "without added sugar," or "no sugar added." This simply means, "We didn't put the sugar in, God did." Again, reading the number of carbohydrates on the nutrition information label is the most accurate way to know the amount of sugar in the product.

16. Understand Fiber

Fiber is the part of a plant your body can't digest, which comes in the form of both water-soluble fiber (which dissolves in water) and water-insoluble fiber (which does not dissolve in water but instead absorbs water); this is what's meant by soluble and insoluble fiber.

Soluble versus Insoluble Fiber

Soluble and insoluble fiber do differ, but they are equally good. Soluble fiber somehow lowers the "bad" cholesterol, or LDL, in your body. Experts aren't entirely sure how soluble fiber works its magic, but one popular theory is that it gets mixed into the bile the liver secretes and forms a type of gel that traps the building blocks of cholesterol, thus lowering your LDL levels. It's akin to a spider trapping smaller insects in its web. Sources of soluble fiber include oats or oat bran, legumes (dried beans and peas), some seeds, carrots, oranges, bananas, and other fruits. Soybeans are also a good source of soluble fiber. Studies show that people with very high cholesterol levels have the most to gain from eating soybeans. Soybeans are also a source of *phytoestrogens* (plant estrogens) that are believed to lower the risks of estrogen-related cancers (for example, breast cancer), as well as lower the incidence of estrogen-loss symptoms associated with menopause.

Whole-grain breads are also good sources of insoluble fiber (flax bread is particularly good because flaxseeds are a source of soluble fiber, too). The problem is understanding what is truly whole grain. For example, there is an assumption that because bread is dark or brown, it's more nutritious; this isn't so. In fact, many brown breads are simply enriched white breads dyed with molasses. (Enriched means that nutrients lost during processing have been replaced.) High-fiber pita breads and bagels are available, but you have to search for them.

17. Understand Psychological Reasons for Weight Gain

At least 80 percent of women at risk for cardiovascular problems weigh 20 percent more than they should for their height and age—the technical definition of obese. But when women go to their doctors or nutritionists, they are given meal plans, lists of what and what not to eat, and so on. The problem is much deeper than simply eating too much food. The key to losing weight for many women is to examine *why* they became obese in the first place.

Many obese women say that they've "dieted themselves up" to their present weight. Obesity is the strongest risk factor for developing cardiovascular problems and common over-fifty cancers, such as colon or breast, as well as Type

2 diabetes. Basically, the longer you've been obese, the more you are at risk. Amazingly, experts have noted that when you lose just 5 pounds, your body actually begins to work more efficiently. The advice to "eat sensibly and exercise," however, just doesn't hold any power for most women battling their own weight issues. Part of the story of Western obesity is understanding where the modern diet came from. After all, you didn't create the modern diet; you were born into it. In fact, the word *diet* comes from the Greek *diatta*, meaning "way of life."

Many European countries experienced a significant drop in a number of obesity-related diseases during the first and second world wars, when meat, dairy foods, and eggs became scarce for a large portion of the population. Wartime rations forced people to survive on brown bread, oats and barley meal, and home-grown produce.

Had it not been for the Depression, we may indeed have seen an increase in obesity-related health difficulties much earlier than we did in North America. The seeds of sedentary life were already planted in the 1920s, as consumer comforts, mainly the automobile and radio, led to more driving, less walking, and more sedentary recreation. The Depression interrupted what was supposed to be prosperous times for everyone. It also intercepted obesity and all diseases related to obesity, as people in many industrialized nations barely ate enough to survive.

The end of World War II marked another significant change in diet: People wanted to celebrate—they gave parties, drank wine. They smoked. They went to restaurants. More than ever before, our diets began to include more high-fat items, refined carbohydrates, sugar, alcohol, and chemical additives. And as women began to manage large families, easy-fix meals in boxes and cans were manufactured in abundance and sold on television to millions. The demand for the diet of leisure radically changed agriculture, too. Today, 80 percent of our grain harvest goes to feed livestock. The rest of our arable land is used for other cash crops such as tomatoes, sugar, coffee, and bananas. Ultimately, cash crops have helped to create the modern Western diet: an obscene amount of meat, eggs, dairy products, sugar, and refined flour.

Since 1940, chemical additives and preservatives in food have risen by 995 percent. In 1959, the Flavor and Extract Manufacturers Association of the United States (FEMA) established a panel of experts to determine the safety status of food flavorings to deal with the overwhelming number of chemicals that companies wanted to add to our foods.

One of the most popular food additives is monosodium glutamate (MSG), the sodium salt of glutamic acid, an amino acid that occurs naturally in protein-containing foods such as meat, fish, milk, and many vegetables. MSG is a flavor enhancer that researchers believe contributes a "fifth taste" to savory foods such as meats, stews, tomatoes, and cheese. It was originally extracted from seaweed and other plant sources to function in foods in the same way as other spices or extracts. Today, MSG is made from starch, corn sugar, or molasses from sugar cane or sugar beets. MSG is produced by a fermentation process similar to that used for making products such as beer, vinegar, and yogurt. While MSG is labeled Generally Recommended As Safe (GRAS) by the FDA, questions about the safety of ingesting MSG have been raised because food sensitivities to the substance have been reported. This fact notwithstanding, the main problem with MSG is that it arouses our appetites even more. Widespread in our food supply, MSG makes food taste better. And the better food tastes, the more we eat.

Hydrolyzed proteins are also used as flavor enhancers. These are made by using enzymes to chemically digest proteins from soymeal, wheat gluten, corn gluten, edible strains of yeast, or other food sources. This process, known as *hydrolysis*, breaks down proteins into their component amino acids. Today, there are several hundred additive substances like these used in our food.

The legacy of the Western diet of leisure is that it has become cheaper to eat out of a box or can than off the land. In the developed Western world, where there's minimum wage, there is also maximum fat. At one time, fat was a sign of prosperity and wealth. Today, wealth is defined by thinness and fitness. Ironically, low-fat foods, diet programs, and fitness clubs attract the segment of our population least affected by obesity. In fact, eating disorders tend to plague women from higher income brackets.

The Coalition for Excess Weight Risk Education, a Washington-based organization comprising the American Diabetes Association, the American Association of Diabetes Educators, the American Society for Clinical Nutrition, the North American Association for the Study of Obesity, and four pharmaceutical manufacturers, issued recent statistics on obesity in the United States. The data can be used to interpret obesity patterns throughout the Western world. Based on a thirty-three-city survey, the National Weight Report found that cities with high unemployment rates and low per capita income tended to have higher rates of obesity. Areas with high annual precipitation rates and a high number of food stores also had greater rates of obesity. (More rainy or snowy days lead to more snacking in front of the television set!)

Why We Like Our Fat

Fat tastes good. Fat also *feels* good in our mouths. Foods that have the particular texture and taste of fat are more acceptable than foods that don't. This is why packaged-good manufacturers describe their products as "smooth, creamy, moist, tender, and rich." All the foods that boast these qualities, from ice cream to chocolate to cheese, give us that unique feeling of satiety and satisfaction that makes us feel good.

Eating is a sensual experience. When we enjoy our food, our brains produce endorphins, "feel-good" hormones that are, ironically, also produced when we exercise. Eating fat is analogous to having a "mouth orgasm." To many of us, without the taste and texture of fat, eating is an empty experience. And when we're in emotional pain or need, the texture and taste of fat become even more important. Bingeing or falling off the diet wagon is not due to losing control but to regaining lost good feelings. Food, as millions of overeaters will tell you, is our friend. It's always there; it never lets us down.

The Impact of Low-Fat Products

Since the late 1970s, Americans have been deluged with low-fat products. In 1990, the United States government launched Healthy People 2000, a campaign to urge manufacturers to double their output of low-fat products by the year 2000. Since 1990, more than a thousand new fat-free or low-fat products have been introduced annually into American supermarkets.

Current guidelines tell us that we should consume less than 30 percent of our calories from fat, while no more than one-third of fat calories should come from saturated fat. According to U.S. estimates, the average person gets between 34 and 37 percent of calories from fat and roughly 12 percent of all calories from saturated fat. Data shows that in terms of "absolute fat," the intake has increased from 81 grams per day in 1980 to 83 grams per day in the 1990s. Total calorie intake has also increased from 1,989 per day in 1980 to 2,153 calories per day. In fact, the only reason that data shows a drop in the percentage of calories from fat is because of the huge increase in calories per day. The result is that we weigh more today than in 1980, despite the fact that roughly ten thousand more low-fat foods are available to us now than in that year.

Most of these low-fat products, however, actually encourage us to eat more. For example, if a bag of regular chips has 9 grams of fat per serving (one serving usually equals about five chips or one handful), you will more likely stick to that one handful. However, if you find a low-fat brand of chips that boasts "50 percent less fat" per serving, you're more likely to eat the whole bag (feeling good about eating "low-fat" chips), which can easily triple your fat intake.

Low-fat or fat-free foods trick our bodies with ingredients that mimic the functions of fat in foods. This is often achieved by using modified fats that are only partially metabolized, if at all, by our bodies. While some foods reduce fat by removing the fat (skim milk, lean cuts of meat), most low fat-foods employ a variety of "fat copycats" to preserve the taste and texture of the food. Water, for example, is often combined with carbohydrates and protein to mimic a particular texture or taste, as is the case with a variety of baked goods or cake mixes. In general, though, the low-fat copycats are carbohydrate based, protein based, or fat based.

Carbohydrate-based ingredients are starches and gums that are often used as thickening agents to create the texture of fat. You'll find these in abundance in low-fat salad dressings, sauces, gravies, frozen desserts, and baked goods. Compared to natural fats, which are about 9 calories per gram, carbohydrate-based ingredients run anywhere from 0 to 4 calories per gram.

Protein-based low-fat ingredients are created by causing the proteins that make them to behave differently. For example, by taking proteins such as whey or egg white, and heating or blending them at high speeds, you can create a creamy texture. Soy and corn proteins are often used in these cases. You'll find these ingredients in low-fat cheese, butter, mayonnaise, salad dressings, frozen dairy desserts, sour cream, and baked goods. They run from 1 to 4 calories per gram.

Low-fat foods that use fat-based ingredients tailor the fat in some way so that we do not absorb or metabolize it fully. These ingredients are found in chocolate, chocolate coatings, margarine, spreads, sour cream, and cheese. You can also use these ingredients as low-fat substitutes for frying foods (you do this when you fry eggs in margarine, for example). Olestra, the new fat substitute just approved by the United States Food and Drug Administration (FDA) is an example of a fat substitute that is not absorbed by our bodies, providing no calories. Caprenin and Salatrim are examples of partially absorbed fats (they contain more long-chain fatty acids; see glossary): These are the more traditional fat-based low-fat ingredients and contain roughly 5 calories per gram.

There's no question that low-fat foods are designed to give you more freedom of choice with your diet, supposedly allowing you to cut your fat without compromising your taste buds. Studies show that "taste" outperforms "nutrition" in your brain. Yet many experts believe that low-fat products create a barrier to weight loss over the long term.

Researchers at the University of Toronto suggest that these products essentially allow us to increase our calories even though we are reducing our overall fat intake. For example, in one study, women who consumed a low-fat breakfast food ate more during the day than women who consumed a higher-fat food at breakfast.

The good news about low-fat or fat-free products is that they are, in fact, lower in fat and are created to substitute for the "bad foods" you know you shouldn't have but cannot live without. The boring phrase "everything in moderation" applies to low-fat products, too. Balancing these products with "good stuff" is the key. A low-fat treat should still be treated like its high-fat original. In other words, don't have double the amount because it's low fat. Instead, have the same amount as you would of the original.

18. Stop Chronic Dieting

The road to obesity is paved with chronic dieting. It is estimated that at least 50 percent of all North American women are dieting at any given time, while one-third of North American dieters initiate a diet at least once a month. The very act of dieting in your teens and twenties can predispose you to obesity later in life. This occurs because most people "crash and burn" instead of eating sensibly. In other words, they're chronic dieters.

The crash-and-burn approach to diet is what we do when we want to lose a specific number of pounds for a particular occasion or outfit. The pattern is to starve for a few days and then eat what we normally do. Or, we eat only certain foods (such as celery and grapefruit) for a number of days and then eat normally after we've lost the weight. Most of these diets do not incorporate exercise, which means that we burn up some of our muscle as well as fat. Then, when we eat normally, we gain only fat. And over the years, that fat simply grows fatter. The bottom line is that when there is more fat on your body than muscle, you cannot burn calories as efficiently. It is muscle that makes it possible to burn calories. Diet it away, and you diet away your ability to burn fat.

If starvation is involved in our trying to lose weight, our bodies become more efficient at getting fat. Starvation triggers an intelligence in the metabolism; the body suddenly thinks it is living in a war zone and goes into "superefficient nomadic mode," not realizing that it is living in modern North America. So, when we return to our normal caloric intake, or even a *lower*-than-normal caloric intake after we've starved ourselves, *we gain more weight.* Our bodies say, "Oh look—food! Better store that as fat for the next famine." Some researchers believe that starvation diets slow down our metabolic rates far below normal so that weight gain becomes more rapid after each starvation episode.

This cycle of crash or starvation dieting is known as the yo-yo diet syndrome, the subject of thousands of articles in women's magazines throughout the last twenty years. Breaking the pattern sounds simple: Combine exercise with a sensible diet. But it's not that easy if you've led a sedentary life most of your adult years. Ninety-five percent of the people who go on a diet gain back the weight they lost, as well as extra weight, within two years. As discussed further on, the failure often lies in psychological and behavioral factors. We have to understand why we need to eat before we can eat less. The best way to break the yo-yo diet pattern is to educate your children early about food habits and appropriate body weight. Experts say that unless you are significantly overweight to begin with or have a medical condition, *don't diet.*

There is another part of the weight story that has do with the role of food and fat in women's lives. Being fat—and/or the overeating behavior that *causes* us to be fat—is perceived by many as a very public rebellion against the role many women are asked to play in this society. So it's important to explore what being fat means to *you*, personally, and the issues surrounding food addiction.

As women, we are the ones that usually do the purchasing and preparing of food for our families. At the same time, we are continuously being deluged with impossible standards of beauty, fitness, and thinness through media images. How do these conflicting roles affect us? For many women, the effect is a feeling of powerlessness. Depending on the woman, by manipulating the body size to be bigger or smaller by eating food or refusing food, we express unconscious desires to achieve more control over our lives.

For the record, compulsive eating is more often a woman's problem, which tells us that it has much more to do with being a woman than doctors and dietitians generally admit. Psychotherapists who specialize in compulsive eating disorders stress that the only way to help women lose weight is to help them understand what conscious or unconscious needs are being met by the fat.

Therapists who work with women about weight loss issues observe that fat isolates a woman, on one hand, and makes her an object of failure, on the other. Women, of course, know this, and *sometimes* use this for psychological advantage. In other words, to the woman, the fat can protect her from being successful in two specific areas: sexual and financial (career-related) endeavors. Many women who are striving for financial success find that a thin body size immediately interferes with that goal. When they are thin, they fear being perceived on sexual terms by male colleagues (or have been so perceived/noticed in the past). They may even fear their *own* sexual desires, or fear being rejected as a sexual object. But when they are fat, they can feel liberated from being perceived as a sexual or "decorative" object and reap the financial rewards of their success nonetheless, or simply enjoy being perceived as productive or competent. By being fat, women can also help to keep their families together by removing themselves from "the market"—avoiding affairs with other men.

On the flip side, many women who have never had success in their lives (sexual or financial) use their fat as a way to remain isolated. This allows them to say to themselves, "If I were thin, I'd be successful." The fatness becomes the reason for failed attempts at personal success, which shields many women from facing their own inner demons and fears, keeping them from the achievements they really want.

For many women, especially those who gained their weight after childbirth, fat has nothing to do with sexuality or personal/financial success. It has to do with their relationship with their mothers, and their own feelings of nurturing and being a mother. After all, it is a mother's breasts that initially nurture us, and it is through our mothers that we learn about food, food behaviors, and so on. Our mothers are also the source of love, comfort, and emotional support. Even when we do not get this from our own personal mothers, we still associate mothering with these emotions. Therapists have observed that body size and eating gets tangled up in mother-daughter relationships and can have varied meanings for the overweight woman. In other words, what your fat says to your mother can mean anything from "I'm a big girl and can look after myself" to "I'm a mess and *can't* look after myself." Some daughters use fat to actually reject the mother's role, or to express anger at their mothers for inadequate nurturing. In some cases, the fat is an unconscious desire to incorporate your mother into your body because she's soothing and nurturing. It's a rather brilliant way of taking your mother with you wherever you go.

Many women find their fat expresses anger at the beauty standard and at the repressive sexual role they're asked to play. The fat is not protection but a deliberate attempt to offend the world. Here, the fat says to the world, "Screw you! If you *really* want to get to know me, then you'll take the time to penetrate my layers. Otherwise, I don't want to know *you!*"

Many women fear being seen. They believe that "the less of me there is, the more people will see;" thus the fat protects the woman from being overexposed emotionally and sexually.

Biological Causes of Obesity

Eating too much high-fat or high-calorie food while remaining sedentary is certainly one biological cause of obesity. Furthermore, a woman's metabolism slows down by 25 percent after menopause, which means that unless she either decreases her calories by 25 percent or increases her activity level by 25 percent to compensate, she will probably gain weight. There are also other hormonal problems that can contribute to obesity, such as an underactive thyroid gland (called hypothyroidism), which is very common in women over age fifty.

Since diet and lifestyle changes are so difficult, there is an interest in finding genetic causes for obesity. If we've inherited obesity, that would mean it is beyond our control, which would probably be comforting for many people. Now that the Human Genome Project is underway, the goal of which is to map every gene in the human body, efforts are proceeding to find the "obesity gene" or "fat gene." Few scientists believe that obesity is *simply* genetic, however. In other words, there are so many environmental and social factors that can "trip" the obesity "switch," finding a specific gene for obesity is about as worthwhile as finding the "anger gene" or "crime gene."

An important theory about why we get fat concerns insulin resistance. It's believed that when the body produces too much insulin, we will eat more to try to maintain a balance. This is why weight gain is often the first symptom of Type 2 diabetes. But then we have to ask, What causes insulin resistance to begin with? Many researchers believe it is triggered by obesity. So it becomes a "chicken or egg" puzzle.

There are also many theories surrounding the function of fat cells. Are some people genetically programmed to have more, or "fatter," fat cells than others? There are no answers here, as yet.

What about the brain and obesity? Some propose that obesity is all in the head and has something to do with the hypothalamus (a part of the brain that controls messages to other parts of the body) somehow malfunctioning when it comes to sending the body the message "I'm full." It's believed that the hypothalamus may control satiation messages. To other researchers, the problem has to do with some sort of defect that prevents the body from recognizing hunger cues or satiation cues; the studies in this area are not conclusive, however.

A study reported in a 1997 issue of *Nature Medicine* showed that people with low levels of the hormone leptin may be prone to weight gain. In this study, people who gained an average of 50 pounds over three years started out with lower leptin levels than people who maintained their weight over the same period. Therefore, this study may form the basis for treating obesity with leptin. Experts speculate that 10 percent of all obesity may be due to leptin resistance. Leptin is made by fat cells and apparently sends messages to the brain about how much fat our bodies are carrying. As with other hormones, it's thought that leptin has a stimulating action that acts as a thermostat of sorts. In mice, adequate amounts of leptin somehow signaled the mouse to become more active and eat less, while too little leptin signaled the mouse to eat more while becoming less active.

Interestingly, Pima Indians in the United States, who are prone to obesity, were shown to have roughly one-third less leptin in blood analyses. Human studies of injecting leptin to treat obesity are in the works right now, but to date have not been shown to be effective.

Drug Treatment for Obesity

Drug treatment for obesity has an awfully shady history. Women have been abused repeatedly by the medical system. Throughout the 1950s, 1960s, and even 1970s, women were prescribed thyroxine, which is thyroid hormone, to speed up their metabolisms. Unless a person has an underactive thyroid gland, or no thyroid gland (which may have been surgically removed), this is a very dangerous medication, which can cause heart failure. Request a thyroid function test before you accept this medication.

Amphetamines or "speed" were often widely peddled to women as well by doctors, but they, too, are dangerous and can put your health at risk.

The U.S. government recently approved an antiobesity pill that blocks the absorption of almost one-third of the fat people eat. One of the side effects of this new prescription drug, called orlistat (brand name Xenical), causes rather embarrassing diarrhea each time you eat fatty foods. To avoid the drug's side effects, simply avoid fat! The pill can also decrease absorption of vitamin D and other important nutrients, however.

Orlistat is the first drug to fight obesity through the intestine instead of the brain. Taken with each meal, it binds to certain pancreatic enzymes to block the digestion of 30 percent of the fat you ingest. How it affects the pancreas in the long term is not known. Combined with a sensible diet, people on orlistat lost more weight than those not on it. This drug is not intended for people who need to lose a few pounds; it is designed for medically obese people. (Orlistat was also found to lower cholesterol, blood pressure, and blood sugar levels.)

One of the most controversial antiobesity therapies was the use of Fenfluramine and phentermine (Fen/Phen). Both drugs were approved for use individually more than twenty years ago, but since 1992, doctors tended to prescribe them together for long-term management of obesity. In 1996, U.S. doctors wrote a total of 18 million monthly prescriptions for Fen/Phen. And many of the prescriptions were issued to people who were not obese. (This is known as off-label prescribing.) In July 1997, the FDA, researchers at the Mayo Clinic, and the Mayo Foundation made a joint announcement warning doctors that Fen/Phen can cause heart disease. On September 15, 1997, Fen was taken off the market. (More bad news has surfaced about Fen/Phen wreaking havoc on serotonin levels, which only reinforces the message that in light of the safety concerns regarding current antiobesity drugs, diet and lifestyle modification are still considered the best pathways to wellness.

A Fen/Phen replacement drug, sibutramine (Meridia), was approved in November 1997 by the FDA. Sibutramine was first developed in the late 1980s as an antidepressant, but like Fen/Phen, it controls appetite by affecting the brain's interpretation of feeling full. Sibutramine differs from Fen/Phen in that it does not interfere with the heart.

Eating Disorders

For 2 percent of the female population in America, starving and purging are considered a normal way to control weight. Only a small number of women are obese because of truly hereditary factors. Most women who think they are overweight are, in fact, at an *ideal* weight for their height and body size. In Western society, the fear of obesity is so crippling that 60 percent of young girls develop distorted body images between grades one and six, believing that they are fat; 70 percent of all women begin dieting between the ages of fourteen and twenty-one. A U.S. study of high school girls found that 53 percent were unhappy with their bodies by age thirteen; and by age eighteen, 78 percent were dissatisfied. The most disturbing fact, revealed in the 1991 critically acclaimed Canadian documentary *The Famine Within,* is that when given a choice, most women *would rather be dead than fat!* Eating disorders are so widespread that abnormal patterns of eating are increasingly accepted in the general population. There are parents who are actually *starving* their young daughters in an effort to keep them thin.

The two most common eating disorders involve starvation. They are *anorexia nervosa* ("loss of appetite due to mental disorder") and bingeing followed by purging, known as *bulimia nervosa.* Women suffering from bulimia will purge after a bingeing episode by inducing vomiting and abusing laxatives, diuretics, and thyroid hormone. The most horrifying examples occur in women with Type 1 diabetes, who sometimes deliberately withhold their insulin to control their weight.

Perhaps the most accepted weight control behavior is overexercising. Today, rigorous, strenuous exercise is used as a method of purging, and has become one of the tenets of socially accepted feminine behavior in the 1990s. A skeleton with biceps is the current ideal.

Women with a history of eating disorders are at much greater risk of developing osteoporosis. Women who are carrying a bit of weight have stronger bones than thin women. Osteoporosis is on the rise in anorexic women as young as age twenty.

Eating disorders are diseases of control that primarily affect women, although more men have become vulnerable in recent years. Bulimics and anorexics are usually over-achievers in other aspects of their lives and view excess weight as an announcement to the world that they are out of control. This view becomes more distorted as time goes on, until the act of eating food in public (in bulimia) or at all (in anorexia) is equivalent to a loss of control.

In anorexia, the person's emotional and sensual desires are perceived through food. These unmet desires are so great that the anorexic fears that once she eats she'll never stop, since her appetite will know no natural boundaries; the fear of food drives the disease.

Most of us find it easier to relate to the bulimic than the anorexic; bulimics express their loss of control through bingeing in the same way that someone else may yell at his or her children. Bulimics then purge to regain their control. There is a feeling of comfort for bulimics in both the binge and the purge. Bulimics are sometimes referred to as "failed anorexics" because they'd starve if they could. Anorexics, however, are masters of control. They never break. I once asked a recovering anorexic the dumb question, "But didn't you get *hungry?*" Her response was that the hunger pangs made her feel powerful. The more intense the hunger, the more powerful she felt; the power actually gave her a high.

When we hear "eating disorder," we usually think about

anorexia or bulimia. There are many people, however, who binge without purging. This is known as binge eating disorder (compulsive overeating). In this case, the bingeing is still an announcement to the world that "I'm out of control." Someone who purges her bingeing behavior is hiding her lack of control. Someone who binges and never purges is *advertising* her lack of control. The purger is passively asking for help; the binger who doesn't purge is aggressively asking for help. It's the same disease with a different result. But there is one more layer when it comes to compulsive overeating, which is considered to be controversial and is often rejected by the overeater: The desire to get fat is often behind the compulsion. Many people who overeat insist that fat is a consequence of eating food, not a *goal*. Many therapists who deal with overeating disagree and believe that if a woman admits that she has an emotional interest in actually being large, she may be much closer to stopping her compulsion to eat.

Furthermore, many women who eat compulsively do not recognize that they are doing so. The following is a typical profile of a compulsive eater:

- Eating when not hungry
- Feeling out of control around food, either trying to resist it or gorging on it
- Spending a lot of time thinking/worrying about food and weight
- Always desperate to try another diet that promises results
- Having feelings of self-loathing and shame
- Hating one's own body

- Being obsessed with what one can or will eat, or *have* eaten
- Eating in secret or with "eating friends"
- Appearing in public to be a professional dieter who's in control
- Buying cakes or pies as "gifts" and having them wrapped to hide the fact that they're for oneself
- Having a pristine kitchen with only the "right" foods
- Feeling either out of control with food (compulsive eating), or imprisoned by it (dieting)
- Feeling temporary relief by not eating
- Looking forward with pleasure and anticipation to the time when one can eat alone
- Feeling unhappy because of eating behavior

Most people eat when they're hungry. But if you're a compulsive eater, hunger cues have nothing to do with when you eat. You may eat for any of the following reasons:

- As a social event: This includes family meals, or meeting friends at restaurants. The point is that you plan food as social entertainment. Most of us do this, but often we do it when we're not even hungry.
- To satisfy mouth hunger—the need to have something in your mouth, even though you are not hungry.
- Eating to prevent *future* hunger: "Better eat now because later, I may not get a chance."
- Eating as a reward for a bad day or bad experience; or to reward yourself for a good day or good experience.

- Eating because "it's the only pleasure I can count on!"

- Eating to quell nerves.

- Eating because you're bored.

- Eating now because you're "going on a diet" tomorrow; hence, the eating is done out of a real fear that you will be deprived later.

- Eating because food is your friend.

Food addiction, like other addictions, can be treated successfully with a twelve-step program. For those of you who aren't familiar with this type of program, I've provided the text of the twelve steps.

The twelve-step program was started in the 1930s by an alcoholic who overcame his addiction by essentially saying, "God, help me!" He found other alcoholics who were in a similar position, and through an organized, nonjudgmental support system, they overcame their addiction by realizing that God—a higher power, spirit, force, physical properties of the universe, or intelligence—*helps those who help themselves.* In other words, you have to want the help. This is the premise of Alcoholics Anonymous (AA)—the most successful recovery program for addicts that exists.

People with other addictions have adopted the same program, using AA and the "The Twelve Steps and Twelve Traditions," the founding literature for AA. Overeaters Anonymous (OA) substitutes the phrase "compulsive overeater" for "alcoholic" and "food" for "alcohol." The theme of all twelve-step programs is best expressed through the Serenity Prayer, the first line being "God grant me the serenity to accept the things I cannot change; the courage to change the things I can; and the wisdom to know the difference." In other words, you can't take back the food you ate yesterday or last year; but you can control the food you eat today instead of feeling guilty about yesterday.

Every twelve-step program also has the twelve traditions, which, essentially, is a code of conduct. To join OA, you need only to take the first step. Abstinence and the next two steps are what most people are able to do in six to twelve months before moving on. In an OA program, abstinence means three meals daily, weighed and measured, with nothing in between except sugar-free or no-calorie beverages and sugar-free gum. Your food is written down and called in. The program also advises you to get your doctor's approval before starting. Abstinence is continued through a one-day-at-a-time process and sponsors—people who call you to check in and who you can call when the cravings hit. Sponsors are recovering overeaters who have been there and who can talk you through your cravings.

OA membership is predominantly female; if you are interested in joining OA and are male, you may feel more comfortable in an all-male group. Many women overeaters overeat because they have been harmed by men, and their anger is often directed at the one male in the room; this may not be a comfortable position if you're a male overeater. For this reason, OA is divided into all-female and all-male groups.

The Twelve Steps of Overeaters Anonymous

Step One: I admit I am powerless over food and that my life has become unmanageable.

Step Two: I've come to believe that a Power greater than myself can restore me to sanity.

Step Three: I've made a decision to turn my will and my life over to the care of a Higher Power, as I understand It.

Step Four: I've made a searching and fearless moral inventory of myself.

Step Five: I've admitted to a Higher Power, to myself, and to another human being the exact nature of my wrongs.

Step Six: I'm entirely ready to have a Higher Power remove all these defects of character.

Step Seven: I've humbly asked a Higher Power to remove my shortcomings.

Step Eight: I've made a list of all persons I have harmed and have become willing to make amends to them all.

Step Nine: I've made direct amends to such people wherever possible, except when to do so would injure them or others.

Step Ten: I've continued to take personal inventory and when I was wrong, promptly admitted it.

Step Eleven: I've sought through prayer and meditation to improve my conscious contact with a Higher Power, as I understand It, praying only for knowledge of Its will for me and the power to carry that out.

Step Twelve: Having had a spiritual awakening as the result of these steps, I've tried to carry this message to compulsive overeaters and to practice these principles in all my affairs.

19. Quick Tips to Trim the Fat

- Whenever you refrigerate foods with animal fat (such as soups, stews, or curry dishes), skim the fat from the top before reheating and serving. A gravy skimmer will also help remove fats; the spout pours from the bottom, and the oils and fats coagulate on top.

- Substitute something else for butter: yogurt (great on potatoes) or low-fat cottage cheese or, at dinner, just dip your bread in olive oil with some garlic, Italian style. For sandwiches, any condiment without butter, margarine, or mayonnaise is fine—mustard, yogurt, and so on.

- Powdered nonfat milk is in vogue again; it is high in calcium, low in fat. Substitute it in any recipe calling for milk or cream.

- Dig out fruit recipes for dessert. Things such as sorbet with low-fat yogurt topping can be elegant. Remember that fruit must be planned for in a diabetes meal plan.

- Season low-fat foods well. That way, you won't miss the flavor fat adds.

- Lower-fat protein comes from vegetable sources (whole grains and bean products); higher-fat proteins come from animal sources.

If you're preparing meat:

- Broil, grill, or boil meat instead of frying, baking, or roasting it. (If you drain fat and cook in water, baking/roasting should be fine.)
- Trim off all visible fat from meat before and after cooking.
- Adding flour, bread crumbs, or other coatings to lean meat adds calories.
- Try substituting low-fat turkey meat for red meat.

Learning to read the fat content in milk is also a good way to cut down:

- Whole milk gets 48 percent of its calories from fat.
- 2% milk gets 37 percent of its calories from fat.
- 1% milk gets 26 percent of its calories from fat.
- Skim milk is completely fat free.
- Cheese gets 50 percent of its calories from fat, unless it's skim milk cheese.
- Butter gets 95 percent of its calories from fat.
- Yogurt gets 15 percent of its calories from fat.

20. Choose a Few Heart-Healthy Herbs

Did you know herbs that are good for the uterus are also good for the heart? Plants that strengthen the uterus and the heart are either green or red, such as hawthorn, rose, strawberry, raspberry, and motherwort. Drinking lots of water, mineral-rich herbal infusions, and fresh grape juice or eating grapes will help you retain fluids and reduce heart palpitations.

To Nourish/Tone the Heart

- Wheat germ oil. One or more tablespoons (15 ml daily).

- Vitamin E oil. One or more tablespoons daily.

- Flaxseed *(Linum usitatissimum)*, also known as linseed, is considered the best heart oil—but only if it is absolutely fresh and taken uncooked. One to 3 teaspoons (5–15 ml) of flaxseed oil first thing in the morning is recommended. You can also grind the seeds and sprinkle them on cereals or salads, or soak flaxseeds in water and drink the whole thing first thing in the morning.

- Other heart-protective oils are the fresh-pressed oils of borage seed or black currant seed.

- Other essential fatty acids can be found in plantain, lamb's quarter, or amaranth.

- Hawthorn berry tincture, 25–40 drops of the berry tincture up to four times a day. Expect results no sooner than six to eight weeks.

- Seaweed.

- Carotene-rich foods. Look for bright-colored fruits and vegetables. The richer the color, the richer they are in carotene.

- Garlic, knoblauch *(Allium sativum)*. Greatest heart benefits come from eating it raw, but you can also purchase deodorized caplets.

- Lemon balm. Steep a handful of fresh leaves in a glass of white wine for an hour or so and drink it with dinner. Or make lemon balm vinegar to use on your salads.

- Dandelion root tincture. Use 10–15 drops with meals.

- Ginseng *(Panax ginseng)*. Chew on the root or use 5–40 drops of tincture.

- Motherwort *(Leonurus cardiaca)*. Use a tincture of the flowering tops, 5–15 drops several times a day as needed.

To Calm the Heart

- Rose flower essence.

- Hawthorn *(Crataegus species)*. Try 25–40 drops up to four times a day. Slow acting, it requires about a month of use before you see results.

- Motherwort tincture. Try 10–20 drops with meals and before bed or 25–50 drops for immediate relief.

- Valerian root, as a tea or tincture.

- Ginger root tea, hot or cold. (May aggravate hot flashes and heavy flows.)

- A piece of real licorice root to slow palpitations.

Blood-Thinning Herbs

Blood thinners, such as aspirin, can reduce the incidence of a stroke or heart attack. A daily spoonful of vinegar made from the leaves, buds, and/or flowers of any of the following herbs can give you the same health benefits as aspirin, but also help calcium absorption and improve your digestion. Do not take blood-thinning herbs if you are bleeding heavily or require surgery.

- Alfalfa
- Birch

- Sweet clover
- Bedstraws
- Poplar
- Red clover
- Willow
- Wintergreen
- Black haw *(Viburnum prunifolium)*, as a tincture. Try a 25-drop dose as needed.

Exercise

21. Understand What Exercise Really Means

The *Oxford Dictionary* defines exercise as "the exertion of muscles, limbs, etc., especially for health's sake; bodily, mental, or spiritual training." In the Western world, we have placed an emphasis on "bodily training" when we talk about exercise, completely ignoring mental and spiritual training. Only recently have Western studies begun to focus on the mental benefits of exercise. (It's been shown, for example, that exercise creates endorphins, hormones that make us feel good.) But we in the West do not encourage meditation or other calming forms of mental and spiritual exercise, which have also been shown to improve well-being and health, particularly in reducing stress—a major risk factor for heart disease.

In the East, for thousands of years, exercise has focused on achieving mental and spiritual health *through* the body, using breathing and postures, for example. Fitness practitioner Karen Faye maintains that posture is extremely important for organ alignment. Standing correctly, with ears over shoulders, and shoulders over hips, with knees slightly bent, and head straight up naturally allows you to pull in your abdomen. According to Faye, many native cultures who balance baskets on their heads or do a lot of physical work with their bodies are noted for correct posture and low rates of osteoporosis.

Nor should we ignore cultural traditions known to improve mental health and well-being, such as traditional dances, active prayers that incorporate physical activity, circles that involve community and communication, and even sweat lodges, believed to help rid the body of toxins through sweating. These are all forms of wellness activities that you should investigate.

22. Understand What Aerobic Means

If you look up the word *aerobic* in the dictionary, what you'll find is the chemistry definition: "living in free oxygen." This is certainly correct; we are all aerobes—beings that require oxygen to live. Some bacteria, for example, are anaerobic; they can exist in an environment without oxygen. All that jumping around and fast movement is done to create faster breathing, so we can take more oxygen into our bodies.

Why are we doing this? Because the blood contains *oxygen!* The faster your blood flows, the more oxygen can flow to your organs. When your health care practitioner tells you to exercise or to take up aerobic exercise, she's not referring solely to increasing oxygen but to exercising the heart muscle. The faster it beats, the better a workout it gets. If you already have heart disease, or on medications that affect your heart, check with your doctor to make sure you are not overworking this vital organ.

Why We Want More Oxygen

When more oxygen is in our bodies, we burn fat (see below), our breathing improves, our blood pressure lowers, and our hearts work better. Oxygen also lowers triglycerides and cholesterol, increasing our high-density lipoproteins (HDL), or the "good" cholesterol, while decreasing our low-density lipoproteins (LDL), or the "bad" cholesterol. This means that your arteries will unclog and you may significantly decrease your risk of heart disease and stroke. More oxygen makes our brains work better, so we feel better. Studies show that depression is decreased when we increase oxygen flow into our bodies. Ancient techniques such as yoga, which specifically improve mental and spiritual well-being, achieve this by combining deep breathing and stretching, which improves oxygen and blood flow to specific parts of the body.

Exercise has been shown to dramatically decrease the incidence of many other diseases, including cancer. Some research suggests that cancer cells tend to thrive in an oxygen-depleted environment. The more oxygen in the bloodstream, the less hospitable you make your body to cancer. In addition, since many cancers are related to fat-soluble toxins, the less fat on your body, the less fat-soluble toxins your body can accumulate.

Burning Fat

The only kind of exercise that will burn fat is aerobic exercise because *oxygen burns fat*. If you were to go to your fridge and pull out some animal fat (chicken skin, red-meat fat, or butter), throw it in the sink, and light it with a match, it will burn. What makes the flame yellow is oxygen; what fuels the fire is the fat. That same process goes on in your body. The oxygen will burn your fat, however you increase the oxygen flow in your body (through jumping around and increasing heart rate or employing an established deep-breathing technique).

The Western Definition of Aerobic

In the West, an exercise is considered aerobic if it makes your heart beat faster than it normally does. When your heart is beating fast, you'll be breathing hard and sweating and will officially be in your target zone or ideal range (the kind of phrases that turn many people off).

There are official calculations you can do to find this target range. For example, it's recommended that by subtracting your age from 220, then multiplying that number by 60 percent, you will find your threshold level—which means, "Your heart should be beating X beats per minute for twenty to thirty minutes." If you multiply the number by 75 percent, you will find your ceiling level—which means, "Your heart should not be beating faster than X beats per minute for twenty to thirty minutes." But this is only an example. If you are on heart medications (drugs that slow your heart down, known as beta-blockers), you'll want to make sure you discuss what target to aim for with your health professional.

Finding Your Pulse

You have pulse points all over your body. The easiest ones to find are those on your neck, at the base of your thumb, just below your earlobe, and on your wrist. To check your heart rate, look at a watch or clock and begin to count your beats for fifteen seconds (if the second hand is on the twelve, count until it reaches fifteen). Then multiply by four to get your pulse.

23. Use the Borg's Rate of Perceived Exertion (RPE)

This is a way of measuring exercise intensity without finding your pulse, and because of its simplicity, it is now the recommended method for judging exertion. This Borg scale, as it's dubbed, goes from 6 to 20. Extremely light activity may rate a 7, for example, while very hard activity may rate a 19. What exercise practitioners recommend is that you do a "talk test" to rate your exertion, as well. If you can't talk without gasping for air, you may be working too hard. You should be able to carry on a normal conversation throughout your activity. What's crucial to remember about RPE is that it is extremely individual; what one person judges a 7, another may judge a 10.

24. Find Other Ways to Increase Oxygen Flow

This will come as welcome news to people who have limited movement due to joint problems, arthritis, or other health complications, ranging from stroke to kidney disease. You can increase the flow of oxygen into your bloodstream without exercising your heart muscle by learning how to breathe deeply through your diaphragm. There are many yoga-like programs and videos available that can teach you this technique, which does not require you to jump around. The benefit is that you increase the oxygen flow into your bloodstream. This is better than doing nothing at all to improve your health and has many health benefits, according to a myriad of wellness practitioners.

25. Start Active Living Instead of Aerobic Living

The term *aerobic activity* means that the *activity* causes your heart to pump harder and faster and causes you to breathe faster, which increases oxygen flow. Activities such as cross-country skiing, walking, hiking, and biking are all aerobic.

But you know what? Exercise practitioners hate the terms *aerobic activity* and *aerobics program* because they are not about what people do in their daily lives. Health promoters are replacing these terms with the phrase *active living*—because that's what becoming nonsedentary is all about. There are many ways you can adopt an active lifestyle. Here are some suggestions:

- If you drive everywhere, pick the parking space farthest away from your destination so you can work some daily walking into your life.

- If you take public transit everywhere, get off one or two stops early so you can walk the rest of the way to your destination.

- Choose stairs over escalators or elevators.

- Park at one side of the mall and then walk to the other.

- Take a stroll after dinner around your neighborhood.

- Volunteer to walk the dog.

- On weekends, go to the zoo or get out to flea markets, garage sales, and so on.

26. Begin Weight-Bearing Activities

You're not just exercising to work your heart muscle and increase oxygen flow, but to make your entire body stronger and more efficient. The side benefit of this is that you can prevent a whole host of health problem, including heart disease. As one fitness expert told me, "If you want a strong house, you need a strong frame." When you increase the load on your bones, your bones increase in mass; similarly, when you decrease the load on your bones, they decrease in mass. And the denser your bones, the harder they are to break or sprain. That's why exercises that build bone mass are important—and you use up calories to boot! By increasing muscular strength through these activities, we also increase flexibility (to help combat falls) and endurance. For example, you'll find that the first time you ride your bike from home to downtown, your legs may feel sore. Do that same ride ten times, and your legs will no longer be sore. That's what's meant by building endurance. Of course, you won't be as out of breath, either, which is another type of endurance.

Hand weights or resistance exercises (using rubber-band gadgets or pushing certain body parts together) help increase what's called lean body mass—body tissue that is not fat. That is why many people find their weight does not drop when they begin to exercise. Leg lifts and arm lifts with weights increase balance, bone strength, and help maintain flexibility. Begin with 1-pound weights and increase slowly to 4 to 5 pounds.

Other forms of resistance exercise involve moving objects or your own body weight to create resistance, using equipment at your gym or fitness center or even common household objects such as water jugs or canned goods. Wearing Velcro weights on your wrists and ankles and just moving around as you normally would is also a good way to increase resistance.

As your muscles become bigger, and your bones become denser, your body fat will decrease. It's recommended that you do weight-bearing exercise four times a week for thirty minutes.

Enjoyable Activities That May Help Build Bone Mass

Try to choose one activity from this list that is your pleasurable sport. If you enjoy your activity, you'll do it more often:

- Walking
- Running
- Jogging
- Bicycling
- Hiking
- Tai chi
- Cross-country skiing
- Gardening
- Weight lifting
- Snowshoeing
- Climbing stairs
- Tennis
- Bowling
- Rowing
- Dancing
- Water workouts

- Badminton
- Basketball
- Volleyball
- Soccer

27. Avoid Hazardous Exercises

Many women find it difficult to just dive into a brand-new fitness routine, particularly if they have certain chronic health problems, such as diabetes, or are taking medications that can affect their hearts. For example, intense exercise in these cases can be dangerous. If you're just beginning to incorporate exercise into your lifestyle after many years of being sedentary, a good plan is to consult with a fitness practitioner in the same way you may consult a nutritionist. Fitness practitioners can be found through your family doctor or through reputable fitness institutions. A fitness practitioner will plan an exercise regimen that is suited to your current physique and shape and will slowly increase the intensity over time, as you build more stamina. Working with a fitness practitioner will also allow you to discuss your health status and any medications you're taking so your activities can complement, rather than aggravate, your health condition.

28. Start Slow

Reports from the United States show that one out of three American adults is overweight, a sign of growing inactivity. Some people are so put off by the health club scene that they become even more sedentary. This is similar to diet failure, where you become so demoralized that you cheated that you binge even more.

What's the definition of sedentary? *Not moving!* If you have a desk job or spend most of your time at a computer, in your car, or watching television (even if it is PBS or CNN), you are a sedentary person. If you do roughly twenty minutes of exercise less than once a week, you're relatively sedentary. You need to incorporate some sort of movement into your daily schedule in order to be considered active. That movement can be anything: aerobic exercise, brisk walks around the block, or walking your dog. If you lead a sedentary lifestyle and are obese, you are at significant risk of developing Type 2 diabetes in your forties, if you are genetically predisposed. If you are not obese, as a woman, your risk is certainly lowered, but you are then predisposed to a number of other problems. If you've been sedentary most of your life, there's nothing wrong with starting off with simple, even leisurely activities such as gardening, feeding the birds in a park, or a few simple stretches. Any step you take toward being more active is a crucial and important one.

Experts also recommend that you find a friend, neighbor, or relative to "get physical" with you. When your exercise plans include someone else, you'll be less apt to cancel them or make excuses for not getting out there.

Things to Do Before "Moving Day"

Choose an activity that's right for you. Whether it's walking, chopping wood, jumping rope, or folk dancing—pick something you enjoy. You don't have to do the same thing each time, either. Vary your routine to avoid monotony. Just make sure that whatever activity you choose is continuous for the duration. Walking for two minutes, then stopping for three isn't continuous. It's also important to choose an activity that doesn't aggravate a preexisting condition, such as eye problems. Lowering your head in a certain way (as in touching your toes) or straining your upper body can increase blood pressure or aggravate eye difficulties. If foot problems are a concern, perhaps an activity that doesn't involve walking, such as canoeing, is better—you get the picture.

- *Choose the frequency.* Decide how often you're going to do this activity. (Two, three, or four times a week? Or once a day?) Try not to let two days pass without doing something. In addition, set a duration goal. If you're elderly or ill, even a few minutes is a good start. If you're sedentary but otherwise healthy, aim for twenty to thirty minutes.

- *Choose the intensity level that's right for you.* This is easy to do if you're using an exercise machine of some kind just by setting the dial. If you're walking, think about how fast you are planning to walk, or how many hills you will be incorporating into your walk. In other words, how fast do you want your heart to beat?

- *Work your activity into your meal plan.* Especially if you are diabetic, once you decide what kind of exercise you'll be doing, and for how long, see your dietitian about working your exercise into your current meal plan. You may need a small snack prior to and after exercise if you're planning to be active longer than thirty minutes. If you are overweight, you do not need to consume extra calories before exercising unless your blood sugar level is low.

- *Tell your doctor what you're doing.* If you have a condition such as diabetes, your doctor may want to monitor your blood sugar more closely (or want you to do so), or adjust your medication. Don't do anything without consulting your doctor first.

29. Choose One Sport

To get started, pick one sport from those listed below. You can vary the activities as you become fit.

More Intense Activities	Less Intense Activities
Skiing	Golf
Running	Bowling
Jogging	Badminton
Stair stepping or stair climbing	Cricket
Trampoline jumping	Swimming
Jumping rope	Sailing
Fitness walking	Strolling
Race walking	Stretching
Aerobics classes	
Roller skating	
Ice skating	
Biking	
Weight-bearing exercises	
Tennis	
Swimming	

30. Try Some of These Variations on Jogging

- After warming up with a fifteen-minute walk, simply walk quickly with maximum exertion for two minutes, then slow down for one minute. Keep your heart rate up on the downhill portion of a walk or a hike by adding lunges or squats.

- Vary the way you walk for coordination and balance. Try lifting the knees as high as you can, as if marching. Alternate with a shuffle, letting the tips of your fingers touch the ground as you walk. Do a sideways "crab" walk. To strengthen the rarely used muscles of the ankles and feet, walk first on the outsides, then on the insides of your feet, or practice walking backwards.

- Use a curb for a step workout, or climb stairs two at a time.

Water Workouts

- Start by walking in water that's relatively shallow (waist or chest deep). Your breathing and heartbeat will let you know how hard you are working. Since you'll be moving fairly slowly, pay attention to your body.

- For all-over leg toning, take fifty steps forward, fifty steps sideways in crablike fashion, fifty steps backward, then fifty steps to the other side.

- To tone your arms, submerge yourself from the neck down, bringing the arms in and out as if clapping. The water will provide natural resistance.

- Deep-water workouts are the most difficult, because every move you make is met with resistance. Wear a flotation vest and run without touching the bottom for optimum exertion and little or no impact.

- You may also want to try buoyant ankle cuffs and Styrofoam dumbbells or kickboards for full-body conditioning in the water.

Deep Breathing

Deep relaxation and yoga breathing, such as alternate nostril breaths, calm the sympathetic nervous system, thus relaxing the small arteries, and permanently lower blood pressure.

Other Risk Factors

31. Find Out If You Have Type 2 Diabetes

If you consume a diet higher in fat than carbohydrates and low in fiber, you increase your risk for Type 2 diabetes if you are genetically predisposed to the disease. If you weigh at least 20 percent more than you should for your height and age (the definition of obese), are sedentary, and over the age of forty-five, you are considered at high risk for Type 2 diabetes. Seventy-three percent of all women with diabetes are obese, and Type 2 diabetes is often called a "heart attack about to happen." Your risk of developing Type 2 diabetes— and cardiovascular complications—further increases if you:

- have high cholesterol or high blood pressure
- smoke
- are of aboriginal descent (this is true for aboriginal peoples all over the world, from Australia to North America; in Canada, First Nations people are at highest risk; in the United States, the Pima Indians are at highest risk)
- are of African or Hispanic descent
- have a family history of Type 2 diabetes
- have a history of gestational diabetes

Impaired Glucose Tolerance (IGT)

Prior to September 1998, many people with Type 2 diabetes were told they had *impaired glucose tolerance* (IGT), which has also been called "borderline diabetes." For the record, there is no such thing as borderline diabetes. And in light of new guidelines, there is no longer any such thing as impaired glucose tolerance, either. But here's what it meant *before* September 1998: IGT was what many doctors referred to as the gray zone between normal blood sugar levels and full-blown diabetes. Normal fasting blood sugar levels (what they are before you've eaten) are between 3 to 5 millimoles (mmol), a unit of measurement that counts molecular volume per liter. In the past, three fasting blood glucose levels between 5 and 7.8 mmol meant that you had IGT. A fasting blood glucose level over 7.8 mmol or a random (any time of day) blood glucose level greater than 11.1 mmol meant that you had diabetes.

That's all changed. Today, anyone with a fasting blood sugar level higher than 7 mmol (determined through a simple blood test) is considered to be in the diabetic rang and is officially diagnosed with Type 2 diabetes.

Signs and Symptoms

If you have any of the symptoms listed below, request to be screened for Type 2 diabetes; this can be done through a simple blood test:

- Weight gain. When your body is not using its insulin properly, you may suffer from excess insulin, which can increase your appetite. This is a classic Type 2 symptom.

- Blurred vision or any change in eyesight (often there is a feeling that your prescription eyewear is weak).

- Drowsiness or *extreme* fatigue at times when you shouldn't be drowsy or tired.

- Frequent infections that are slow to heal. (Women should be on alert for recurring vaginal yeast infections or vaginitis, which means vaginal inflammation, characterized by itching and/or foul-smelling discharge.)

- Tingling or numbness in the hands and feet.

- Gum disease. High blood sugar affects the blood vessels in your mouth, causing inflamed gums; the sugar content can get into your saliva, causing cavities in your teeth.

Diabetes experts also point out the following possible signs of Type 2 diabetes:

- Irregular periods, such as changes in cycle length or flow (this could be a sign of menopause as well)

- Depression, which could be a symptom of either low or high blood sugar

- Headaches (from hypoglycemia)

- Insomnia and/or nightmares (from hypoglycemia)

- Spots on the shin (known as necrobiosis diabeticorum)

- Decaying toenails

- Muscle pains or aches after exercise (high blood sugar can cause lactic acid to build up, which can cause pain that prevents you from continuing exercise)

You may also have diabetes if your doctor has diagnosed you with the following:

- High cholesterol
- High blood pressure
- Anemia
- Cataracts
- Salivary-gland stones

Controlling Your Blood Sugar

Controlling your blood sugar means testing your blood sugar (discuss with your health care practitioner how frequently to test yourself), meal planning (with a dietitian), and exercising. By controlling your blood sugar, you will stay free of the symptoms of diabetes as well as reduce your risk of complications, such as heart disease.

Since heart disease is a major complication of Type 2 diabetes, and postmenopausal women are more prone to heart disease as a result of estrogen loss, the current recommendation is for women with Type 2 diabetes to seriously consider hormone replacement therapy after menopause. Right now, the Women's Health Initiative (WHI) is studying 25,000 postmenopausal women, many of whom have diabetes. The results of this study (expected by 2003) are expected to present concrete facts regarding the perceived benefits of HRT for postmenopausal women with Type 2 diabetes.

Meal Plans

Meal plans recommended by registered dietitians are tailored to your individual goals and medication regimen. Men and women will usually require different quantities of food.

The goal is to keep the supply of glucose consistent by spacing out your meals, snacks, and activity levels accordingly. If you lose weight, this will allow your body to use insulin more effectively, but not all people with Type 2 diabetes need to lose weight. If you're on insulin, meals will have to be timed to match your insulin's peak. A dietitian can be helpful by prescribing an individualized meal plan that addresses your specific needs (weight control, shift work, travel, and so on).

A good meal plan will ensure that you are getting enough nutrients to meet your energy needs and that your food is spread out over the course of the day. For example, if your meal plan allows for three meals with one to two snacks, meals should be spaced four to six hours apart so your body isn't overwhelmed. If you are obese, snacks will likely be discouraged because they can cause you to oversecrete insulin and increase your appetite. A meal plan should also help you to eat consistently rather than bingeing one day and starving the next.

A good meal plan will ensure that you're getting the vitamins and minerals you need without taking supplements, such as iron, calcium, folic acid, vitamins A, B_1, B_2, B_3, C, D, and E. Here are the golden rules of diabetes meal plans:

- Eat three meals a day at fairly regular times (spaced four to six hours apart).
- Ask your dietitian to help you plan your snacks.
- Try to eat a variety of foods each day from all food groups.
- Learn how to gauge serving sizes, volume of bowls and glasses, and so on.

- Ask your dietitian or diabetes educator about how to adjust your diet if you're traveling (this depends on whether you take medication, where you're going, what foods will be available, and so on).

- Draw up a "sick-day plan" with your dietitian. This will depend on what your regular meal plan includes.

- Ask about any meal supplements, such as breakfast bars, sports bars, or meal replacement drinks. How will these figure into your meal plan?

- Choose lower-fat foods more often.

32. Understand What High Blood Pressure (Hypertension) Means

About 12 percent of North American adults suffer from hypertension, or high blood pressure. What is blood pressure? The blood flows from the heart into the arteries (blood vessels), pressing against the artery walls. The simplest way to explain this is to think about a liquid-soap dispenser. When you want soap, you need to pump it out by pressing down on the little dispenser pump, the "heart" of the dispenser. The liquid soap is the "blood" and the little tube, through which the soap flows, is the "artery." The pressure that's exerted on the wall of the tube is therefore the "blood pressure."

When the tube is hollow and clean, you needn't pump very hard to get the soap; it comes out easily. But when the tubing in your dispenser gets narrower as a result of old, hardened, gunky liquid soap blocking the tube, you have to pump down much harder to get any soap, while the force the soap exerts against the tube is increased. Obviously, this is a simplistic explanation of a very complex problem, but essentially, the narrowing of the arteries, created by higher blood pressure, forces your heart to work harder to pump the blood. If this goes on too long, your heart muscle enlarges and becomes weaker, which can lead to a heart attack. Higher pressure can also weaken the walls of your blood vessels, which can cause a stroke.

The term *hypertension* refers to the tension or force exerted on your artery walls. (*Hyper* means "too much," as in "too much tension.") Blood pressure is measured in two readings: X over Y. The X is the systolic pressure, which is the pressure that occurs during the heart's contraction. The Y is the diastolic pressure, which is the pressure that occurs when the heart rests between contractions. In "liquid soap" terms, the systolic pressure occurs when you press the pump down; the diastolic pressure occurs when you release your hand from the pump and allow it to rise back to its "resting" position.

Normal blood pressure readings are 120 over 80 (120/80). Readings of 140/90 or higher are generally considered borderline, although for some people this is still a normal reading. For the general population, 140/90 is "lecture time," when your doctor will begin to counsel you about dietary and lifestyle habits. By 160/100, many people are prescribed an antihypertension drug, which is designed to lower blood pressure.

The most common causes of high blood pressure are obesity, inactivity, and stress. High blood pressure is also exacerbated by tobacco and alcohol consumption and too much sodium or salt in the diet. (People of African descent tend to be particularly salt sensitive.)

If high blood pressure runs in the family, you're considered at greater risk of developing hypertension. High blood pressure can also be caused by kidney disorders (which may be initially caused by diabetes) or pregnancy (known as pregnancy-induced hypertension). Medications are also common culprits. Estrogen-containing medications (such as oral contraceptives), nonsteroidal anti-inflammatory drugs (NSAIDs) such as ibuprofen, nasal decongestants, cold remedies, appetite suppressants, certain antidepressants, and other drugs can all increase blood pressure. Be sure to check with your pharmacist.

The Role of Stress

Hypertension and heart disease are also believed to be triggered by stress. Before you can look at what you can do to manage your stress, the first order of business is understanding what, exactly, stress is. Generally, stress is defined as a negative emotional experience associated with biological changes that allow you to adapt to it. In response to stress, your adrenal glands pump out stress hormones that speed up your body—your heart rate increases and your blood sugar levels increase so that glucose can be diverted to your muscles in case you have to run. This is known as the fight-or-flight response.

The problem with stress hormones in the twenty-first century is that the fight-or-flight response isn't usually necessary, since most of our stress is emotional. Occasionally, we may want to flee from a bank robbery or mugger, but most of us just want to flee from our jobs or our kids! In other words, our stress hormones actually put a physical strain on our bodies and can lower our resistance to disease, which can impact the body from head to toe. We can suffer from these stress-related difficulties:

- Headaches
- Gastrointestinal problems
- Bladder problems
- Heart problems
- Back pain
- High blood pressure (predisposing us, of course, to heart disease)
- High cholesterol (possibly predisposing us to heart disease)

Good Stress

Good things come from good stress, even though it feels stressful or bad in the short term. Stress challenges us to stretch ourselves beyond our capabilities, which is what makes us meet deadlines, "push the envelope," and invent creative solutions to our problems. Examples of good stress include challenging projects; positive life-changing events (moving, changing jobs, or ending unhealthy relationships); confronting fears, illness, or people who make us feel bad (this is one of those "bad in the short term/good in the long term" situations). Essentially, whenever a stressful event triggers emotional, intellectual, or spiritual growth, it is a good stress. It is often not the event as much as it is your *response* to the event that determines whether it is a good or bad stress. The death of a loved one can sometimes lead to personal growth because we may see something about ourselves we did not see before—new resilience, for example. So even a death can be a good stress, though we grieve and are sad in the short run.

Bad Stress

Bad stress results from boredom and stagnation. When no growth occurs from the stressful event, it is bad stress. When negative events don't seem to yield anything positive in the long run, the stress can lead to chronic and debilitating health problems. This is not to say that we can't get sick from good stress, either, but when there is nothing positive from the stress, it has a much more negative effect on our health. Some examples of bad stress include stagnant jobs or relationships, disability from terrible accidents or diseases, or long-term unemployment. These kinds of situations can lead to depression, low self-esteem, and a host of physical illnesses.

Managing Stress

What we perceive as stressful has great bearing on how well we manage it. Women that are already overloaded will feel stress more keenly as well. In general, we feel stress when we experience:

- Negative events
- Uncontrollable or unpredictable events
- Ambiguous events (versus clear-cut situations)

How stressed you become has much to do with your personality as well. For example, if you have a negative outlook on life, you'll probably feel more stress than someone with a positive attitude. Some women like to find meaning in uncontrollable events, which gives them a sense of control. Others like the challenge of difficult situations.

Our strategies for coping also vary. Some women like to avoid the stress and minimize the problem. This has short-term benefits but, over the long term, the stress does not disappear. Women who confront the stress right away will feel more anxious at first, but will probably feel relief in the long run when they have dealt with it. People who suffer fewer stress-related health problems use humor, spiritual support, and social networking to deal with stress.

If the following statements sound like you, you're probably not managing stress very well:

- I tend to imagine all the terrible things that could possibly happen to me rather than just concerning myself with the stressful situation at hand.

- I stop what I'm doing and devote all my energy toward fixing the problem immediately. (I might as well do this because if I don't, I will just drive myself crazy with worry.)

- I relive my latest crisis in my mind over and over again, even after it's been solved.

- I actually picture the stressful situation in my mind's eye, as well as picturing the worst possible outcome.

- I get the feeling that I'm losing control over everything.

- I experience a sinking feeling in my stomach, my mouth getting dry, my heart pounding, or my neck and shoulder muscles tightening.

- I have trouble falling asleep at night and wake up in the middle of the night.

- I tend to make mountains out of molehills (I sort of know I'm doing this, but I can't stop myself).

- I have difficulty speaking or notice my hands or fingers trembling.

- I notice my thoughts racing.

Stress reduction depends entirely on the source of your stress. The only way to control stress that is beyond your control is to modify your response to it. For many women, this takes time and may require some work with a qualified counselor. If you are the source of your own stress because you're too hard on yourself, or are a perfectionist, you need to work on lowering your self-expectations and forgiving yourself for not being perfect. Again, working with a therapist or counselor may help. In the meantime, here are a few suggestions for reducing some sources of daily stress:

- Isolate the exact source of stress and see if there's a solution. (Taking the time to think about what, in fact, the real problem is can work wonders.)

- See the humor in difficult situations, and try to look at lessons learned instead of beating yourself up.

- When times get tough, surround yourself with supportive people: close friends, family members, and so on.

- Don't take things so personally. When people don't respond to you the way you'd like, consider other factors. For instance, maybe the other person has problems unrelated to you that are affecting his behavior.

- Focus on something pleasant in the future, such as a vacation, and allow yourself time to daydream, plan, and so on.

- Just say no. If you can't take on that small favor or extra task, just politely say "I'd love to, but it's impossible."

- Take time out for yourself. Spend some time alone and block everyone out once a week or so. This is a great opportunity to just go for a long walk and get in a little exercise.

- Make lists. Some people find list making really helps; others find it is just another chore in and of itself. But if you haven't been a list maker, try it. It might help you get a little more organized and focused on the tasks at hand.

- Look at some alternative healing systems, perhaps massage or Chinese exercises, such as qi gong (pronounced "chi kong") or tai chi.

- Eat properly.

Finding a Good Stress Counselor or Therapist

When you are hunting for a counselor to work with you on reducing stress, any of the following professionals can help:

- *Psychiatrist:* This is a medical doctor who specializes in the medical treatment of mental illness and is able to prescribe drugs. Many psychiatrists also do psychotherapy, but this isn't always the case. The appropriate credentials should read: Jane Doe, M.D. (medical doctor), F.A.C.P. (Fellow, American College of Physicians). (Or, in Canada, F.R.C.P. [Fellow, Royal College of Physicians].) That means this doctor has gone through four years of medical school and has completed a residency program in psychiatry, which, depending on the state, lasted approximately four years, and is registered in the American College of Physicians and Surgeons. (Or, if trained in Canada or the United Kingdom, the Royal College of Physicians and Surgeons.)

- *Psychologist or Psychological Associate:* This is someone who can be licensed to practice therapy with either a master's degree or a doctoral degree. Clinical psychologists have a master of science degree (M.Sc.) or master of arts degree (M.A.) and will usually work in a hospital or clinic setting. They are often found in private practice as well. Clinical psychologists can also hold a Ph.D. (doctor of philosophy) in psychology, an Ed.D. (doctor of education), or, if they're American, a Psy.D. (doctor of psychology), a common degree in the United States. Psychologists often perform testing and assessments and plan treatments. They can also do psychotherapy, may have hospital admitting privileges, and should be registered with their state licensing board. Licensure is required in all fifty states. Licensure requirements are generally uniform across states, authorizing the psychologist to independently diagnose and treat mental and nervous disorders on completion of both a doctoral degree in psychology (Ph.D., Psy.D., or Ed.D.) and a minimum of two years of supervised experience in direct clinical service. In some states, psychologists can also prescribe drugs.

- *Social Worker:* This professional holds a BSW degree (bachelor of social work) and/or a MSW degree (master of social work), having completed a bachelor's degree in another discipline (which is not at all uncommon). Some social workers have Ph.D.s as well. A professional social worker holds a degree in social work and meets state legal requirements. The designation CSW stands for Certified Social Worker. It is a legal title granted by the state. A designation of

ACSW refers to the National Association of Social Worker's (NASW) own nongovernmental national credential and stands for Academy of Certified Social Workers. Unlike the CSW, which in addition to the exam requires graduation (in most states) from a master's level program, the ACSW requires two years of supervised experience following graduation from such a program. Some social workers have a "P" and "R" in their titles; these letters stand for CSWs who have become qualified under state law to receive insurance reimbursement for outpatient services to clients with group health insurance. Each initial refers to different types of insurance policies. The "P" requires three years of supervised experience, while the "R" requires six years.

- *Psychiatric Nurse:* This is most likely a registered nurse (R.N.) with a bachelor of science in nursing (B.Sc.) (which isn't absolutely required) who probably, but not necessarily, has a master's degree in nursing, too. The master's degree could be either an M.A. (master of arts) or an M.Sc. (master of science). This nurse has done most of her training in a psychiatric setting and may be trained to do psychotherapy.

- *Counselor:* This professional has usually completed certification courses in counseling and therefore has obtained a license to practice psychotherapy; she may have a university degree (but this is not required). Frequently, though, counselors will have a master's degree in a related field, such as social work. Or, they may have a master's degree in a field having nothing to do with mental health. The term *professional counselor* is used to represent those persons who have earned a minimum of a master's degree and posseses professional knowledge and demonstrable skills in the application of mental health, psychological, and human development principles in order to facilitate human development and adjustment throughout the life span. As of January 1999, the District of Columbia and forty-four states have enacted some type of counselor credentialing law that regulates the use of titles related to the counseling profession. The letters "CPC" stand for Certified Professional Counselor and refer to the title granted by the state legislative process. The letters "LPC" stand for Licensed Professional Counselor and refer to the most often granted state statutory counselor credential. No matter what letters you see, however, it's always a good idea to ask your counselor what training she has had in the field of mental health.

- *Marriage and Family Counselor:* This is somewhat different than the broader term *counselor.* This professional has completed rigorous training through certification courses in family therapy and relationship dynamics and has obtained a license to practice psychotherapy. This professional should have the designations MFT or AAFMT in his title. MFTs have graduate training (a master's or doctoral degree) in marriage and family therapy and at least two years of clinical experience. Forty-one states currently license, certify, or regulate MFTs.

It's important to discuss fees with your therapist up front, so you know what services are covered by your health plan. In general, mental health services in hospitals are covered by insurance, as are services provided by psychiatrists. But social workers or counselors in private practice are all fee for service. Call the National Association of Social Workers (NASW) at 800-638-8799 to determine what a social worker or counselor in private practice should be charging and to obtain a copy of the NASW Code of Ethics. If you want to see someone in private practice, but can't afford the fees, some community-provided counseling services are based on your ability to pay. Experts consulted for this book concurred that it is considered bad practice for a counselor to agree to see someone who cannot (or will not) pay for her services. The counselor is offering a service, not a charity, and the professional relationship should be respected. As of this writing, psychiatrists typically charge roughly $100 to $175 per hour/session, clinical psychologists charge roughly $85 to $120 per hour/session, while social workers charge $65 to $110 per hour/session.

If you have health insurance through a managed care plan, you may be in for a rude awakening when it comes to coverage of psychiatric services. Most plans cover only thirty days of inpatient psychiatric care per year and twenty outpatient visits to a psychotherapist. This is fine if you require only short-term therapy, but this coverage is inadequate for most people suffering from depression or mood disorders. Some plans offer conversion of benefits, meaning that you can convert your thirty days of inpatient coverage to thirty extra days of outpatient visits, giving you fifty outpatient visits covered.

An extremely important consideration for anyone having psychiatric services covered by a health insurance plan is confidentiality. Managed care companies require frequent record reviews by psychiatric services providers, which

means that confidentiality between you and your mental
health care provider may be compromised. Discuss this
aspect of treatment when you discuss fees and costs; it's
important.

Going for a Test Drive

Okay. You found someone you think is qualified to be your
therapist. That doesn't mean you found the right therapist
for *you*. Ask yourself the following questions when you first
sit down with this therapist. If you find you answer no to
many of the questions below, you should ask yourself
whether you're really with the right professional. There is
no magic number of no's here, but these questions will help
you gauge how you truly feel about this therapist.

1. Is this someone with whom you feel comfortable?

2. Is this someone you can trust?

3. Is this someone with whom you feel calm?

4. Is this someone who makes you feel safe?

5. Does this person respect you (or treat you with
   respect)?

6. Does this person seem flexible?

7. Does this person seem reliable?

8. Does this person seem supportive?

9. Does this person have a supervisor or mentor with
   whom she consults on difficult or challenging cases?

33. Learn How to Lower Your Blood Pressure Without Drugs

There are some effective steps you can take to lower your blood pressure yourself:

- Change your diet and begin exercising (see Diet and Exercise sections).
- Limit alcohol consumption to no more than 2 oz. of liquor or 8 oz. of wine or 24 oz. of beer per day, or even less for liver health.
- Limit your salt intake to about 1½ teaspoons per day. Cut out all foods high in sodium, such as canned soups, pickles, soy sauce, and so on. Some canned soups contain 1,000 mg of sodium, for example. That's a lot!
- Increase your intake of calcium or dairy products and potassium foods (for example, bananas). Some still-unproven research suggests that people with hypertension are calcium and potassium deficient.
- Lower your stress levels. Studies show that when you reduce your stress response, your blood pressure decreases.

Herbs to Lower Blood Pressure

The following herbs can help to lower blood pressure:

- Hawthorn tincture. 10–20 drops three times daily
- Motherwort tincture. 10–20 drops three times daily
- Dandelion root tincture. Use 10–15 drops with meals
- Potassium. 80–85 percent of people who eat six portions of potassium-rich foods daily will reduce

their need for blood pressure–lowering medication by half or more

- Raw garlic. Just one-half to one clove of raw garlic a day can dramatically reduce your blood pressure; mince it raw into a variety of dishes, including eggs, rice, or potatoes
- Ginseng
- Seaweed

34. Discuss Blood Pressure–Lowering Drugs with Your Doctor

If you can't lower your blood pressure through lifestyle changes, you may be a candidate for some of the following blood pressure–lowering drugs:

- *Diuretics.* Diuretics are the most commonly used blood pressure medication. Also known as water pills, diuretics work by flushing excess water and salt (often 2 to 4 pounds worth!) out of your system. But diuretics may actually increase the risk of heart attack by leaching potassium salts needed by the heart; the heart may respond to blocked nerve signals by trying harder and harder, until it fails. Another common side effect of diuretic therapy is low potassium. Levels of potassium tend to drop when diuretics replace the low-fat diet you've worked so hard to maintain. If you make sure not to substitute one therapy for another, diuretics will not affect your potassium levels. Other side effects include increased blood sugar and cholesterol levels.

- *Beta-blockers.* Beta-blockers alter the way hormones such as adrenaline control blood pressure. They slow down the heart rate by decreasing the strength of the heart's contractions. Beta-blockers are most often used by young people or people with coronary artery disease. Possible side effects include fatigue and an increase in blood sugar and cholesterol levels.

- *Centrally acting agents.* These drugs act through centers in the brain to slow the heart rate and relax the blood vessels. Possible side effects include stuffy nose, dry mouth, and drowsiness.

- *Vasodilators.* Vasodilators dilate, or relax, the blood vessels, thereby reducing blood pressure.

- *ACE inhibitors.* ACE inhibitors lower blood pressure by preventing the formation of a hormone called angiotensin II, which causes the blood vessels to narrow. ACE inhibitors are also used to treat heart failure. Possible side effects include cough and swelling of the face and tongue.

- *Alpha-blocking agents.* Alpha-blocking agents block the effects of noradrenaline, allowing the blood vessels to relax. Blood pressure decreases with treatment, as does cholesterol. You may also notice an increase in HDL, or "good" cholesterol. A possible side effect is blood pressure variation when standing versus reclining.

- *Calcium-channel blockers.* Calcium-channel blockers limit the amount of calcium entering the cells, allowing the muscles in the blood vessels to relax. Possible side effects include ankle swelling, flushing, constipation, and indigestion.

35. Be Aware of the High-Cholesterol Controversy

Cholesterol is a whitish, waxy fat made in vast quantities by the liver. That's why liver and other organ meats are high in cholesterol! Cholesterol is needed to make hormones as well as cell membranes. If you have high cholesterol, the excess cholesterol in your blood can cause narrowed arteries, which can lead to a heart attack. Saturated fat, discussed in detail in the Diet section, is often a culprit when it comes to high cholesterol because it causes your body to produce its own cholesterol. The highest levels of cholesterol, however, are due to a genetic defect in the liver. The story of women and high cholesterol is still unfolding. You see, when it comes to high cholesterol, newer research is showing that it is not as much of a risk factor for heart disease in women as it is for men. If you've already suffered a heart attack, then following a low-saturated-fat diet will help to lower the "bad cholesterol" (the LDL or low-density lipoproteins) and raise your HDL (high-density lipoproteins, or "good cholesterol"). Similarly, if you smoke, have high blood pressure, are obese, have Type 2 diabetes, or have a family history of heart disease, following the low-fat, lower-cholesterol diet will help improve your health, too.

For healthy women over age sixty-five with higher than normal cholesterol, though, who don't smoke and who have no other risk factors for heart disease other than age, there's no clear benefit to lowering cholesterol, or even worrying about it. We know, for example, that very few premenopausal women with high cholesterol ever develop heart disease, leading researchers to conclude that other factors are more significant for women than high cholesterol. So, while high cholesterol is definitely linked to male heart disease, it is *not* definitely linked to female heart disease and, in fact, may not even be a big deal. Most physicians will recommend a low-fat diet to women with other risk factors for heart disease because it can't hurt and will improve other health problems. That said, there are clinical practice guidelines that physicians follow when managing a woman's cholesterol (see number 36).

36. Know the Guidelines for Managing Your Cholesterol

The current guidelines most physicians in North America follow when managing cholesterol in women encourage women over age twenty to begin a lower-cholesterol diet (see numbers 11 through 20) if their cholesterol levels are 200 mg/dl or more. If you have very low "good" or HDL cholesterol levels (less than 35 mg/dl), then your doctor should measure the "bad" or LDL cholesterol levels; an LDL level below 130 mg/dl is desirable. LDL levels of 130–159 mg/dl are borderline high. Levels of 160 mg/dl or above are high. A low-saturated-fat diet will probably be recommended. If you already have heart disease, you should aim to have LDL readings of about 100 mg/dl or less, lower than the guidelines for women without heart disease. In this case, your doctor may recommend that, in addition to a low-saturated-fat diet, you also take a cholesterol-lowering drug (see number 39).

Cholesterol levels are checked through a simple blood test. You can also ask your pharmacist about the availability of home cholesterol tests.

If your blood cholesterol is between 200 and 239 mg/dl, so long as you don't smoke, are not obese, have normal blood pressure, are premenopausal, and do not have a family history of heart disease—you're fine! A high total cholesterol reading should always be followed up with an HDL/LDL analysis.

37. Know How to Lower Cholesterol Without Drugs

By modifying your diet (see numbers 11 through 20) and exercising (see numbers 21 through 30), you'll probably be able to lower your cholesterol without taking any medication. Vitamin E has been shown to lower cholesterol, too, preventing the formation of arterial plaque. A 46 percent drop in the incidence of heart attack was reported in a study of 87,000 nurses taking vitamin E. On the basis of that study, doctors now recommend a dosage of 100 IU (international units) daily. As for vitamin C, we still don't know how much vitamin C is needed to reduce the risk of heart attack. Consumption of large amounts of vitamin C was associated with lower rates of coronary artery disease in an eight-year study at Brigham and Women's Hospital in Boston.

38. Have Some Wine

Alcohol has been proven to raise your good cholesterol (HDL). This fact was discovered in the late 1980s when researchers investigated why the French, who ate such rich food, had very low rates of heart disease. It was the wine; red wine, in particular, was shown to decrease the risk of cardiovascular disease. So wine can be beneficial, so long as you drink it in moderation.

Many women are also concerned about the calories they take in when they have that wine. So here's the deal: A glass of dry wine with your meal adds about 100 calories. Half soda water and half wine (a spritzer) contains half the calories. When you cook with wine, the alcohol evaporates, leaving only the flavor.

If you're a beer drinker, you're basically having some corn, barley, and a couple of teaspoons of malt sugar (maltose) when you have a bottle of beer. The corn and barley ferment into mostly alcohol and some maltose. Calorie-wise, that's about 150 calories per bottle plus 3 teaspoons of malt sugar. A light beer has fewer calories but still contains at least 100 calories per bottle.

The stiffer the drink, the fatter it gets. Hard liquors such as scotch, rye, gin, and rum are made from cereal grains; vodka, the Russian staple, is made from potatoes. In this case, the grains ferment into alcohol. Hard liquor averages about 40 percent alcohol, but has no sugar. Nevertheless, you're looking at about 100 calories per small shot glass, so long as you don't add fruit juice, tomato or Clamato juice, or sugary soft drinks.

39. Ask About Cholesterol-Lowering Drugs

For many, losing weight and modifying fat intake simply aren't enough to bring cholesterol down to optimal levels. You may be a candidate for one of the numerous cholesterol-lowering drugs that have hit the market in recent years. These medications, when combined with a low-fat, low-cholesterol diet, target the intestine, blocking food absorption, and/or the liver, where they interfere with the processing of cholesterol. These are strong drugs, however, and ought to be a last resort after really giving a low-fat, low-cholesterol diet a chance. You might be given a combination of cholesterol-lowering medications to try along with a low-cholesterol diet. It's important to ask about all side effects accompanying your medication because these can include gastrointestinal problems, allergic reactions, blood disorders, and depression. One study looking at male patients taking cholesterol-lowering drugs found an unusually high rate of suicide and accidental trauma. There have not been enough studies on women taking these drugs to truly know how they interact with women's health conditions. At any rate, here's what's available as of this writing. Please note that only the generic drug names are listed:

- *Niacin.* When taken properly, niacin is the best cholesterol treatment available. In 1986, the Coronary Drug Project (a National Institutes of Health study) found that prolonged use of niacin significantly reduced mortality rates among heart attack victims. It has since become one of the most popular cholesterol-lowering drugs on the market. Niacin, a water-soluble B vitamin, can lower LDL by 30 percent and triglyceride levels by as much as 55 percent. It also increases HDL by about 35 percent. Also known as nicotinic acid, niacin must be taken in large doses (1–3 mg/day) in order to be effective. Because the dosage is up to seventy-six times higher than the recommended daily allowance, side effects are common. Many patients experience itching, flushing, and panic attacks. Switching to slow-release capsules, taking an aspirin thirty minutes before taking the medication, or taking it on a full stomach might help alleviate some of these symptoms. Niacin can aggravate both stomach ulcers and diabetes.

- *Statins.* Statins such as Mevacor and Zocor hinder the liver's ability to produce cholesterol, keeping LDL levels to a minimum while increasing levels of HDL. When combined with the proper diet, statins can reduce your risk of death from heart disease by as much as 40 percent. However, certain lovastatins (Zocor) have been known to cause liver damage, muscle pain, and weakness.

- *Cholestyramine.* Cholestyramine helps the body eliminate cholesterol through the gut. It is considered the safest of the cholesterol-lowering drugs; it has also been around the longest. A National Institutes of Health study in the early 1980s demonstrated that cholestyramine decreases heart attack deaths by lowering cholesterol levels. In fact, for each 1 percent drop in the cholesterol levels of participants, there was a 2 percent drop in death rates. Pretty impressive when you consider the fact that the average decline in blood cholesterol was 25 percent. Although cholestyramine reduces LDL or bad cholesterol, it can sometimes raise triglyceride levels. It can also trigger a host of side effects, the most unpleasant of which is *really bad* gas. Cholestyramine interferes with the effectiveness of digitalis, diuretics, warfarin, fat-soluble vitamins, and beta-blockers. It can also lead to gallstones. Cholestyramine should be taken in the morning and at bedtime.

- *Gemfibrozil.* Gemfibrozil lowers cholesterol and triglyceride levels in the blood. The rate of coronary artery disease among 4,000 men with high cholesterol involved in a Finnish study of this drug dropped 34 percent. Gemfibrozil should be take in 600 mg tablets twice daily.

- *Arginine.* Preliminary studies suggest that this amino acid may lower cholesterol levels and improve coronary blood flow by acting as an antioxidant and maintaining elasticity in blood vessel tissues. Arginine is currently available without a prescription.

- *Coenzyme Q10.* Japanese and European practitioners love this powerful antioxidant, but more studies are needed to prove its reputed effect on arterial plaque.

40. Practice Safe Sex and Get Checked for Chlamydia

Although this sounds crazy, it's actually true: People with heart disease have much higher rates of infection with chlamydia, a sexually transmitted disease that is particularly rampant in women aged eighteen to thirty-five. The chlamydia/heart disease connection surfaced in 1996, with a startling study published in the *Journal of the American College of Cardiology.* The results indicated that people with diseased arteries were infected with chlamydia at dramatically higher rates than those with normal arteries. This study showed that 79 percent of those with diseased arteries tested positive for chlamydia infection, compared to 4 percent of the control patients examined, which confirmed smaller studies that were done earlier throughout Europe. These are such dramatic findings that it is now considered good practice for all women to be screened for chlamydia not just for their sexual health, but their heart health, too. What it all boils down to is that preventing heart disease in women may involve using condoms.

Chlamydia was discovered in the late 1970s and is neither a typical bacteria nor a virus. It is very small, like a virus in size, and has some characteristics of a bacteria, but it can't manufacture its own energy the way a bacteria or virus can. Instead, it acts like a parasite, entering cells and using *their* energy. It is caused by a bacterium known as *Chlamydia trachomatis*, but because it falls into this murky "no man's land" of odd behavior, chlamydia is not always easy to detect. Ten percent of the time, people who have chlamydia will test negative for it. Chlamydia is one of the most common STDs in North America right now, and in the sexually active crowd aged eighteen to thirty, 50 percent have chlamydia. Chlamydia is particularly nasty, however, because it is usually *asymptomatic* (meaning no symptoms). In one year, about four and a half million women in North America will be infected with chlamydia, and 60 percent of them will not have any symptoms. Aside from the heart disease connection, the disease can also do a lot of damage in other ways.

Some experts estimate that chlamydia causes 50 percent of all pelvic infections and 25 percent of all tubal pregnancies, due to scarring of the fallopian tubes. It can also cause urethral infections, cervicitis (inflammation of the cervix), and pelvic inflammatory disease (PID), which can lead to subsequent infertility or complications during pregnancy or birth.

The symptoms of early-stage chlamydia are usually nonexistent for four out of five women. The most common symptom, if any, is increased or abnormal vaginal discharge, which usually develops about fourteen days after infection. Sometimes there is a strong, rather foul vaginal odor that develops as well. Painful urination, unusual vaginal bleeding, bleeding after sex, and low abdominal pain may also be signs, and the cervix may be inflamed (noticeable when examined by a doctor). If your cervix bleeds easily after a Pap smear, this is also a major clue. If chlamydia spreads to your uterus and fallopian tubes, it will have progressed to PID.

The best thing you can do if you're sexually active is to be regularly screened for chlamydia by your family doctor; the test is 90 percent accurate. The screening is simple: Your doctor takes a culture swab of cervical mucus. It can be done in conjunction with a Pap test. How regularly should you be swabbed? Every time you have a new partner.

The good news about chlamydia is that it is *extremely* easy to treat: Tetracycline will cure it. It is also believed that hormonal contraceptives increase your risks of exposure because the cervical mucus changes and is therefore a better host for chlamydia.

A Review of Safe Sex

Think you're too old to read this? Think again. As women age, the vaginal lining thins, making older women more vulnerable to STDs such as chlamydia and, worse, HIV. So here's a review of some wise practices. Safe sex refers to an entire array of sensible, health-conscious practices, which *include but are not limited to using condoms.* Safe sex includes the following:

1. *Abstinence.* Never sleep with someone you don't know. Abstain from intercourse until the relationship is serious.

2. *Ask the difficult questions.* Get to know your partner well. Ask about sexual history, anal sex, and intravenous drug use, and ask to see proof of a negative HIV test (volunteer to take the test as well).

3. *Never have sex without using both a latex condom and spermicide unless you and your partner are monogamous and have both tested negative for HIV infection.* Don't fall for lines like "All of my relationships have been monogamous," or "I don't fool around." Be sure. Basically, unless you've been with the same person for over two years, know for a fact that he's *never* strayed, and know for a fact that he *is* HIV-negative, don't have sex without a latex condom and spermicide. It is believed that spermicide helps kill the HIV virus.

4. *Never perform oral sex without a barrier unless you and your partner are monogamous and have both tested negative for HIV infection.* HIV is transferred through semen, vaginal secretions, or menstrual blood. You don't want to swallow it. And, gums frequently bleed, especially if there is vigorous thrusting in the mouth.

5. *Carry latex condoms and spermicide with you at all times.*

6. *Abstain from all sexual contact during a menstrual period.* That semen-to-blood contact is a real killer. Even if you're using condoms, you don't want to risk "double trouble."

7. *Abstain from all sexual activity during a vaginal infection.* Vaginal discharge can be more infectious to the male during this time; HIV is more easily transferred to women through this kind of vaginal discharge.

8. *Never have sex before you're ready.*

9. *Never engage in anal sex without the use of two condoms and plenty of lubricant.* Public health professionals warn that for a heterosexual couple, the risks associated with anal intercourse *may* outweigh the pleasures. First, penetration causes tearing of rectal tissue and bleeding. *This is why HIV can so easily be transmitted during unprotected anal sex. It provides direct semen-to-blood contact.* Worse, the tears in your rectum are aggravated by bowel movements. This can mean permanent damage to your bowels and rectal tissue and pain and bleeding when you have a bowel movement. During unprotected anal sex, a male can get feces on his penis, and then transfer fecal material into the vagina. This is bad news and can introduce a whole gamut of nasty bacteria into your vagina. If you *must* have anal sex, here are the rules:

- *Use two condoms and plenty of proper lubricant.* The lubricant will moisten the orifice and help to prevent the tearing of rectal tissue. Two condoms are necessary in case one condom breaks.

- *Never use Vaseline or petroleum jelly as a sexual lubricant.* It can erode the condom and cause it to break or dissolve inside the rectum (or vagina). Use a proper sexual lubricant, such as KY Jelly.

- *After anal intercourse, make sure your partner carefully washes and dries his penis and then his hands, and puts on a fresh condom before continuing with further activity.* You'll want to make sure that no fecal material is transferred into your vagina and that no blood from your rectal tears gets inside your vagina.

- *After anal intercourse, reapply lubricant into your rectum to help soothe any irritation that results.*

- *If you're engaging in regular anal intercourse, make sure you have a full "STD sweep" twice a year, and ask for a rectal exam as well.* If anal sex is only a one-time occurrence, go for an exam after that experience. Report any bleeding, pains, or difficult bowel movements you have after the incident.

- *If you're having anal intercourse, make sure you inform your doctor.* Anal intercourse may affect the results of your exam. It's important your doctor knows you're engaging in it so she can accurately analyze the results of your exams and further advise you on safer sex practices.

10. *Never share needles.* Although taking narcotics intravenously was always unhealthy, and sharing dirty needles carried all kinds of germs and infections including hepatitis B, until AIDS the obvious risks associated with this kind of behavior were ignored by drug abusers. If you're an IV drug user, here are the rules:

- *Always use clean needles; never share your needles; never use someone else's needles.* There are needle exchange programs set up all over the continent. Ask your doctor about where you can go to make sure you're getting clean needles.

- *If you're taking drugs intravenously for legitimate health reasons, make sure you have regular checkups with your family doctor, and make sure you're using a screened blood product.* Don't use any product unless you know for a fact it's been screened for HIV infection.

- *As a rule, get an AIDS test done once a year (or ask your doctor to recommend reasonable time intervals) to make sure you haven't been exposed.* HIV can remain dormant for several years before it becomes active.

Just because you've had one negative AIDS test doesn't mean you weren't exposed to HIV. As an IV drug user, you are in the highest risk category for developing AIDS. So keep testing until you're absolutely sure.

- *Avoid having sex with an intravenous drug user; if you must, use two condoms and plenty of spermicide.* If you are the drug user, always disclose your drug use to your partner, and if you can't abstain from sex, insist on two spermicidal condoms.

What's Safest Sex?

Here is a list of sexual activities, the safest activities first. The further down the list, the riskier the activity!

- No sex/abstinence
- Fantasy
- Voyeurism
- Exhibitionism
- Masturbation
- Massage
- Hugging
- Vibrators or other sex toys (not shared)
- Dry kissing
- Body to body rubbing or "tribadism" when fluids are not involved
- Mutual masturbation
- Mutual masturbation with clean sex toys
- Wet kissing

- Shared hand/genital contact with a barrier
- Oral sex with a dental dam (female to female; male to female) and/or condom
- Oral sex with no semen
- Vaginal intercourse with a latex condom (either male condom or female condom)
- Anal sex with a condom
- Fisting with a barrier
- Shared hand or finger/genital contact with cuts or sores
- Oral sex without a barrier during menstruation
- Fisting without a barrier such as a glove
- Oral/anal contact without a barrier
- Oral sex with semen and/or no condom
- Anal sex with no semen and no condom
- Anal sex with semen and no condom
- Sharing needles of any kind

Hormone Replacement Therapy

41. Understand the Connection Between Menopause and Heart Disease

Menopause is a Greek term taken from the words *menos*, which means "month," and *pause*, which means "arrest" — the arrest of the menstrual cycle. It is a time in every woman's life when her ovaries are slowing down, running out of eggs, and getting ready to retire.

Natural menopause and *menarche* (the first menstrual period) have a lot in common—they are both *gradual* processes into which women ease slowly. A woman doesn't suddenly wake up to find herself in menopause any more than a young girl wakes up to find herself in puberty. However, when menopause occurs *surgically*—the by-product of an oopherectomy, ovarian failure following a hysterectomy, or certain cancer therapies—it can be an extremely jarring process. *One out of every three women in North America will not make it to the age of sixty with her uterus intact.* These women may indeed wake up one morning to find themselves in menopause and, as a result, will suffer far more noticeable and severe menopausal symptoms than their counterparts experiencing natural menopause. It is because of *surgical* menopause that *hormonal replacement therapy* (HRT) and *estrogen replacement therapy* (ERT or unopposed estrogen)

117

have become such hotly debated issues in women's health. The loss of estrogen, in particular, leads to drastic changes in the body's chemistry that trigger a more aggressive aging process, including predisposing women to heart disease.

Estrogen loss increases *all* women's risk of heart disease, which is the major cause of death for postmenopausal women. If you have other risk factors, such as Type 2 diabetes, for example, the risk of heart disease is two to three times higher than in the general female population.

The average American woman will live until age seventy-eight, meaning that she will live one-third of her life after menopause. Many women, of course, will also be concerned about their risk of breast cancer. Taking estrogen can stimulate or trigger the growth of an estrogen-dependent breast cancer cell (that is, a breast cancer cell that "feeds" or thrives on the hormone estrogen). Current studies show that this type of cancer is far more treatable than other kinds of breast cancers. And, as I'll discuss in the last item of this book, since many more women die from heart attacks than breast cancer—particularly if they have other risk factors—the trade-off of preventing heart disease (or even fractures from osteoporosis) must be considered as a benefit.

42. Know When You're in Menopause

Socially, the word *menopause* refers to a process, not a precise moment in the life of your menstrual cycle. Medically, the word *menopause* does *indeed* refer to one precise moment: the date of your last period. The events preceding and following menopause amount to a huge change for women both physically and socially, however. Physically, this process is divided into four stages:

- *Premenopause.* Although some doctors may refer to a thirty-two-year-old woman in her childbearing years as premenopausal, this is not really an appropriate label. The term *premenopause* ideally refers to women on the cusp of menopause. Their periods have just *started* to get irregular, but they do not yet experience any classic menopausal symptoms such as hot flashes or vaginal dryness. A woman in premenopause is usually in her mid- to late forties. If your doctor tells you that you're premenopausal, you might want to ask her how she is using this term.

- *Perimenopause.* This term refers to women who are in the thick of menopause—their cycles are wildly erratic, and they are experiencing hot flashes and vaginal dryness. This label is applicable for about four years, covering the first two years prior to the official last period to the two years following the last menstrual period. Women who are perimenopausal will be aged from the mid- to late forties to about fifty-one.

- *Menopause.* This term refers to your final menstrual period. You will not be able to pinpoint your final period until you've been completely free from periods for one year. Then, you count back to the last period you charted, and *tha*t date is the date of your menopause. *Important: After more than one year of no menstrual periods, any vaginal bleeding is now considered abnormal.*

- *Postmenopause.* This term refers to the last third of most women's lives. It describes women ranging from those who have been free of menstrual periods for at least four years to women celebrating their one hundredth birthdays. Once you're past menopause, you'll be referred to as postmenopausal for the rest of your life.

Sometimes, the terms *postmenopausal* and *perimenopausal* are used interchangeably, but this is technically inaccurate.

"Diagnosing" Premenopause or Perimenopause

When you begin to notice the signs of menopause, either you'll suspect the approach of menopause on your own, or your doctor will put two and two together when you report your "bizarre" symptoms. There are two very simple tests that will accurately determine what's going on, and what stage of menopause you're in. Levels of follicle stimulating hormone (FSH) dramatically rise as menopause begins; these levels are easily checked using one blood test. (Normally, FSH "kick-starts" the menstrual cycle and signals the ovaries to release an egg, known in the early parts of the cycle as a follicle; the levels of FSH rise as the ovaries start to slow down.) In addition, your vaginal walls will thin, and the cells lining the vagina will not contain as much estrogen. Your doctor will take a Pap-like smear from your vaginal walls—simple and painless—and then analyze the smear to check for vaginal atrophy—the thinning and drying out of your vagina. In addition, as I'll discuss below, you need to keep track of your periods and chart them as they become irregular. Your menstrual pattern will be an additional clue to your doctor about whether you're pre- or perimenopausal.

Signs of Natural Menopause

In the past, a long list of hysterical symptoms have been attributed to the "change of life," but medically there are really just three classic *short-term* symptoms of menopause: erratic periods, hot flashes, and vaginal dryness. All three of these symptoms are caused by a decrease in estrogen. As for the emotional symptoms of menopause, such as irritability, mood swings, melancholy, and so on, they are actually caused by a *rise in FSH*. As the cycle changes and the ovaries' egg supply dwindles, FSH is secreted in very high amounts and reaches a lifetime peak, as much as fifteen times higher than before; this is the body's way of trying to "jump-start" the ovarian engine. This is why the urine of menopausal women is used to produce human menopausal gonadotropin (HMG), the potent fertility drug that consists of pure FSH.

Decreased levels of estrogen can make you more vulnerable to stress, depression, and anxiety because estrogen loss affects REM sleep. When we're less rested, we're less able to cope with stresses that normally may not affect us.

Watch for these two key signs or changes:

Erratic periods. Every woman will begin to experience irregular cycles before her last period. Cycles may become longer or shorter, with extended bouts of amennorhea. There will also be flow changes; periods may suddenly become light and scanty, or very heavy and crampy.

Hot flashes. Roughly 85 percent of all pre- and perimenopausal women experience what are known as hot flashes. They can begin when periods are still regular, or when they have just started to become irregular. The hot flashes usually stop between one and two years after your final menstrual period. A hot flash can feel different for each woman. Some women experience a feeling of warmth in their faces and upper bodies; some women feel hot flashes as simultaneous sweating and chills. Some women feel anxious, tense, dizzy, or nauseated just before the hot flash; others feel tingling in their fingers or heart palpitations just before. Some women experience hot flashes during the day; others experience them at night, and may wake up so wet from perspiration that they need to change their bedsheets or night clothes. Nobody really understands what causes a hot flash, but researchers believe that it has to do with mixed signals from the hypothalamus, which controls both body temperature and sex hormones. Normally, when the body is too warm, the hypothalamus sends a chemical message to the heart to cool off the body by pumping more blood, causing the blood vessels under the skin to dilate, which makes you perspire. During menopause, however, it's believed that the hypothalamus gets confused and sends this cooling-off signal at the wrong times. A hot flash is not the same as being overheated. Although the skin temperature often rises between 4 and 8 degrees Fahrenheit, the internal body temperature drops, creating this odd sensation. Why does the hypothalamus get so confused? It's because of decreasing levels of estrogen. We know this because when synthetic estrogen is given to replace natural estrogen in the body, hot flashes disappear. Some researchers believe that a decrease in luteinizing hormone (LH) is also a key factor, and a variety of other hormones that influence body temperature are being looked at as well. Although hot flashes are harmless in terms of health risks, they are disquieting and stressful. Certain groups of women will experience more severe hot flashes than others:

- *Women who are in surgical menopause.*
- *Women who are thin.* When there's less fat on the body to store estrogen reserves, estrogen loss symptoms are more severe.
- *Women who don't sweat easily.* An ability to sweat makes extreme temperatures easier to tolerate. Women who have trouble sweating may experience more severe flashes.

43. Know the Difference Between HRT and Natural Hormone Replacement Therapy (NHRT)

Many of you may have heard the media hype surrounding natural hormone replacement therapy (NHRT) (which includes natural progesterone) versus conventional hormone replacement therapy (HRT). The difference is akin to breast milk versus formula for a baby. NHRT is a combination of human estrogens and natural human progesterone. HRT, on the other hand, is a factory-made estrogen, much of which is derived from horse estrogen, and a factory-made progesterone, called progestin. Now, many reports and studies show that the symptoms of menopause are better controlled with NHRT, resulting in fewer side effects. Studies also show that the benefits of HRT—protection from heart disease and osteoporosis—are more dramatic and pronounced using NHRT.

What NHRT Contains

When you go on NHRT, you're getting about 60 to 80 percent estriol, 10 to 20 percent estrone, and 10 to 20 percent estradiol, as well as natural human progesterone and DHEA (dehydroepiandrosterone), a natural androgen, which turns into a natural testosterone in the body (something all women need to maintain their sex drive). On HRT, you're getting 75 to 80 percent estrone, 6 to 15 percent equilin (a horse-derived estrogen), and about 5 to 19 percent estradiol, as well as a factory-made progesterone and sometimes anabolic steroids if your libido needs a boost.

The bottom line is that human women do better with human hormones rather than animal-derived hormones, just as human infants do better on human milk than cow's milk. As you can see from the range of concentrations of various natural estrogens, however, it may take a while for you to find just the right dose of each kind of natural estrogen and progesterone. You have to work with your doctor and experiment until you get it right. There is a perception out there that NHRT is perfect the first time you take it, but many women have to tinker with their triple estrogens before they find the right combination for them. A typical starting prescription for NHRT is 10 percent estrone, 10 percent estradiol, and 80 percent estriol, mixed with about 25 to 30 mg of natural progesterone and 10 to 30 mg DHEA, which should (but doesn't always) convert into necessary amounts of testosterone. (If it doesn't, you may need to add a steroid to the mix of natural hormones if your libido is very low, as mentioned previously.)

Where Do You Find NHRT?

All the books and articles about natural hormone therapy can mislead you into thinking that it is available everywhere. This is not so. You can't just walk into a health food store and buy natural estrogens or progesterones. They need to be prescribed by a doctor (although the doctor need not be an M.D.; many naturopathic doctors prescribe them, too). A pharmacist must be trained to prepare a doctor's prescription for NHRT from scratch. This person is known as a compounding pharmacist. Not all pharmacies are compounding pharmacies, so ask your doctor or current pharmacist about where to get a prescription prepared. You can also call the International Academy of Compounding Pharmacists (IACP) or the Professional Compounding Centers of America, Inc. (PCCA), for the nearest compounding pharmacist in your area. Many compounding pharmacists are members of either or both organizations. You can reach the PCCA at 1-800-331-2498 or at www. compassnet.com/~iacp/.

44. Know the Benefits of Hormone Therapy

Whether you choose natural or synthetic hormones (N)HRT is a prophylactic therapy and a cure for the menopausal symptoms. These hormones are designed to replace the estrogen lost after menopause, and hence prevent or even reverse the long-term consequences of estrogen loss, such as heart disease, osteoporosis, skin changes, vaginal thinning and dryness, and other ailments. (N)HRT is also designed to treat the short-term symptoms of menopause, such as the hot flashes and vaginal dryness.

Therefore, you have the choice of taking (N)HRT as either a *short-term therapy* or a *long-term therapy*. There are also some risks involved with HRT and ERT that you'll need to weigh against the benefits, however.

Heart Benefits

In addition to protecting our bones and maintaining our reproductive organs, estrogen also helps to maintain appropriate levels of high-density lipoproteins (HDL), which keep our arteries clear of plaque, preventing them from clogging and causing heart attacks and strokes. By raising HDL, known as the "good cholesterol," the "bad" cholesterol—low-density lipoproteins that cause fatty substances to collect in the arteries, causing arteriosclerosis—drops. Estrogen also helps protect us from rheumatoid arthritis. It's our ovaries, of course that make estrogen, but other sources of estrogen come from androstenedione (a hormone) and testosterone, which are converted by our tissues into a form of estrogen called *estrone,* a weaker form of estrogen than the kind our ovaries produce. Obese women have estrone in greater amounts. Although this may prevent severe menopausal symptoms, estrone is *not* considered a potent enough form of estrogen to protect against osteoporosis or heart disease.

Today, all women who have gone through menopause naturally and who decide to go on (N)HRT will be given estrogen *and* progesterone. The progesterone, of course, triggers the uterine lining to shed regularly, which prevents the risk of endometrial cancer, associated with unopposed estrogen therapy—only estrogen and no progesterone, which was what women used to be given. Estrogen and progesterone *together* also mirror the normal menstrual cycle and help prevent the side effects normally felt with estrogen alone. (If you've had a hysterectomy, you won't need any progesterone; you're not at risk for uterine cancer since your uterus is gone.)

What to Expect in the Short Term

Generally, (N)HRT will begin to relieve your estrogen-loss menopausal symptoms within days of starting the therapy. Your hot flashes will disappear, your vagina will become moist again and will lubricate on its own during sex, and your vagina's acidic environment will be restored, preventing yeast and other vaginal infections from plaguing you. However, if you change your mind and go *off* the therapy, your symptoms will return in a far more severe form!

The heart benefits seen with estrogen only arise if the estrogen is taken orally, not in patches or vaginal creams.

In order for estrogen to work its magic with HDL, it needs to be metabolized in the liver.

Estrogen, however, will not counteract a poor diet and lifestyle. If you smoke, drink excessively, are under tremendous stress, or eat copious amounts of the wrong foods (you know the ones), don't expect estrogen alone to shield you from heart disease.

45. Understand How to Take Conventional HRT or ERT

Since many women opt for factory-made, or conventional, HRT, it's important to know how to take it. The most common estrogen product is called Premarin. Premarin uses a synthesis of various estrogens that are derived from the urine of pregnant horses, to make the estrogen mimic nature more accurately. Premarin literally stands for "pregnant mare's urine"—from "pre" (pregnant), "mar" (mare's), and "in" (urine). Premarin is a trade name for this type of replacement estrogen and comes in pills, patches, and vaginal creams. Other common synthetic forms of estrogen include micronized estradiol, ethinyl estradiol, esterified estrogen, and quinestrol.

For short-term therapy, you may only need the vaginal cream to help with vaginal dryness or bladder problems. For long-term therapy, you'll need the pill form if you want to protect yourself from heart disease. The drugs in Premarin come in a variety of other brand names, each just as good as the other. Estrogen can also be worn; it's placed in a small plastic patch about the size of a silver dollar, worn on the abdomen, thighs, or buttocks, and changed twice weekly.

When estrogen is in patch or cream form, it goes directly to the bloodstream, bypassing the liver, and hence does not affect HDL, or protect against heart disease. Some women also have an allergic reaction to the skin patch and break out in a rash. If you're one of them, try taking estrogen in other forms.

Progesterone

Synthetic progestins (a family of progesterone drugs that include natural progesterone) are norethindrone or norethindrone acetate. Natural progestin is medroxyprogesterone.

Progestins are taken in separate tablets along with estrogen. Together, the estrogen and progestin you take is called HRT. HRT can be administered two ways: *cyclically* or *continuously*. Taking HRT cyclically is very similar to taking an oral contraceptive because the hormones closely mirror a natural cycle. The first day you start is considered day 1 of your mock cycle. You take estrogen from days 1 to 25; you then add the progesterone from days 14 to 25. Then you stop all pills and bleed for two or three days—just as you would on a combination oral contraceptive. This vaginal bleeding is called *withdrawal bleeding*. It is lighter and shorter than a normal menstrual period, lasting only two or three days—just like a period on a combination birth control pill. In fact, if the bleeding is heavy or prolonged, this is a warning that something's not right, and you should get it checked.

In addition, you may experience breakthrough bleeding—spotting during the first three weeks after you begin HRT. This kind of bleeding is also similar to what happens on a combination oral contraceptive. It usually goes away after a few months, but you should report it anyway. You may need to switch to a lower dose of estrogen or take a higher dose of progestin. Once your mini-period of withdrawal bleeding is finished, you simply start the cycle again. Many women can't tolerate cyclical HRT because they feel they should be *rid* of their periods by now and not have to deal with pads and tampons ever again. However, it is believed that cyclical HRT offers slightly better heart protection.

When HRT is taken continuously, you simply take one estrogen pill and one progestin pill each day. When you do it this way, the progesterone *counteracts* the estrogen; no uterine lining is built up, so no withdrawal bleeding needs to happen.

Appropriate Dosages

Every woman requires a different dosage of estrogen and progestin. You will always be placed on the *lowest* possible dosage of either one at first; the dosage may be increased gradually if necessary. If your estrogen dosage is too high, you'll experience side effects similar to those seen with estrogen oral contraceptives: headaches, bloating, and so on.

Before you determine how much estrogen you'll need, it's crucial to first assess how much your body is still producing; this really depends on your weight, menopausal symptoms, and a hundred other things.

Estrogen

Estrogen tablets come in dosages of 0.3 mg, 0.625 mg, 0.9 mg, or 1.25 mg. Dosages also depend on why you're taking estrogen. For women at high risk for osteoporosis, the most common starting dosage is 0.625 mg. But for women who just want short-term relief from menopausal symptoms, such as hot flashes, starting at 0.3 mg is more usual. If you forget to take your estrogen tablet one day, don't worry about it. You will not need to double up the way you would with birth control pills. It's important, however, that once you begin the estrogen, you continue to take it daily without a significant break (such as more than two days). Studies show that when you stop taking estrogen, you may suffer from far more severe hot flashes and insomnia than you did before you started it.

If instead of taking estrogen orally, you are using the vaginal estrogen cream, you can use the cream for about three weeks on and one week off. Women who opt for the vaginal cream have decided on estrogen for short-term relief of vaginal dryness and thinning, as well as from urinary incontinence, another postmenopausal problem, discussed below. Vaginal cream does not, however, relieve hot flashes or offer any protection from osteoporosis or heart disease. Using vaginal creams occasionally, the way you would use lubricant, for example, will do you no good. Again, every woman is different, as are brands and dosage measurements for each brand. Make sure you discuss how much estrogen you're getting per application with either your doctor or your pharmacist.

As for skin patches, they contain either 4 or 8 mg of estrogen. The 4 mg patch releases .05 mg of estrogen daily; the 8 mg patch releases twice that amount. You'll need to change the patch twice a week. Some doctors recommend that you wear the patch for three weeks, and then take a one-week break from it before you start again. Obviously, you'll need to discuss this with your doctor and decide what's right for you. Again, women who take the patch will not derive any heart benefits, but they will be protected from bone loss and menopausal symptoms. In fact, the patch delivers a more continuous flow of estrogen than pills because there is no fluctuation in terms of dosage. With pills, it's impossible to be as consistent with when you take your pill; there is human error involved.

The Androgen Strain

ERT or HRT sometimes contains androgens, male hormones. Doctors prescribe androgens to improve your libido, if you're experiencing problems in that regard. This may indeed be appropriate, but it's important to *know what you're getting!* If your androgen dosage is too high, you can develop male features, such as increased body hair, a deeper voice, and shrinking breasts. These symptoms do not magically vanish once you go off the androgens. Some studies also show that added androgens may have a negative effect on blood cholesterol, actually *increasing* heart disease risk. This may explain why men taking estrogen derive no HDL benefits.

46. Know the Side Effects of Conventional HRT

If you're taking *cyclical* progestins with your estrogen because you still have your uterus, bleeding is *not* a side effect! The whole point of adding progestin to your estrogen is to trigger withdrawal bleeding and allow your uterine lining to be routinely shed. If you're taking continuous progestins with your estrogen, bleeding is not the norm and should be investigated.

A common side effect of estrogen is fluid retention because estrogen decreases the amount of salt and water excreted by the kidneys; when this is retained in the body, legs, breasts, and feet can swell. Because of the fluid retention, you may weigh more.

Nausea is another common side effect, also seen with oral contraceptives. This happens during the first two or three months of therapy, and should disappear on its own. Some women find that taking their pills at night relieves this. Decreasing the dosage is also an option.

Some other side effects reported include headaches, skin color changes called *melasma* on the face (similar to those in pregnancy), heavy cervical mucous secretion, liquid secretion from the breasts, change in curvature of the cornea, jaundice, loss of scalp hair, and itchiness. Again, these side effects vary and depend on the brand you're taking, the dosage, your medical history, and so on. Many women suffer no side effects at all. Finally, a minor side effect estrogen causes is vitamin B_6 deficiency, as seen with oral contraceptive use. Symptoms of this deficiency are vague and include fatigue, depression, loss of concentration, loss of libido, and insomnia. These problems are easily remedied by taking a vitamin B_6 supplement.

47. Know When to Say No to Conventional HRT

Conventional HRT or ERT is not for everyone. Some women make better candidates than others. Here's a guide that may help you make the decision:

- *Are you in a high-risk group for heart attacks or strokes?*
  If so, ERT or HRT will lower your risk.

- *Are you in a high-risk category for endometrial cancer?*
  If so, taking progestin to trigger withdrawal bleeding will lower your risk.

- *Are you in a high-risk group for developing osteoporosis?* Again, ERT or HRT will lower your risk.

- *Do you have a history of breast cancer?* You shouldn't be on either ERT or HRT if you have a history of breast cancer.

- *Have you had a stroke?* Neither ERT nor HRT is recommended.

- *Do you have a blood clotting disorder?* Neither ERT nor HRT is recommended.

- *Do you have undiagnosed vaginal bleeding?* Neither therapy is recommended.

- *Do you have liver dysfunction?* You can be on the estrogen patch or vaginal cream to relieve your menopausal symptoms but you shouldn't take any pills.

You should think twice about HRT or ERT if you have any of the following disorders:

- Sickle cell disease
- High blood pressure
- Migraines
- Uterine fibroids
- A history of benign breast conditions such as cysts or fibroadenomas
- Endometriosis
- Seizures
- Gallbladder disease
- A family history of breast cancer
- A past or current history of smoking

At a quick glance, here's a summary of HRT's benefits:

- Reduces bone loss during and after menopause.
- Reduces menopausal symptoms.
- Reduces the risk of heart disease by 40 to 50 percent (benefits are less clear when progesterone is added to the estrogen; some studies suggest this may even cancel out the protection against heart disease).
- Reduces thinning of vaginal tissue and associated discomforts.

At a quick glance, here's a summary of HRT's risks:

- It is not effective for every woman.
- It can raise cholesterol levels.
- Side effects of depression and anxiety have been reported.
- In women with a high risk of breast cancer, or a history of severe blood clotting disorders, it can increase the risk.

48. Consider Phytoestrogens

If you are uncomfortable with the idea of taking hormone replacement therapy, you may wish to consider the therapeutic benefits of phytoestrogens, or plant estrogens. Many women are treating their menopausal symptoms with capsules of powdered herbs, such as licorice, burdock, wild yam, motherwort, and dong quai *(Angelica sinensis)*.

These herbs contain a multitude of chemicals, including estrogenic substances. Although phytoestrogens have been used in Asian cultures for centuries to treat hot flashes, they're just beginning to catch on in the West. The first controlled trial began in 1996 at Columbia-Presbyterian Medical Center in New York.

Many food sources such as tofu and other soy foods contain high concentrations of phytoestrogens. Scientists believe this may account for the incredible lack of menopausal symptoms in Japan, which has a soy-heavy diet. Blood levels of phytoestrogens are ten to forty times higher in Japanese women than in their Western counterparts, and Japanese women report hot flashes about one-sixth as often as Western women. Even most vegetarians do not consume nearly as much soy as the average Japanese woman.

More interesting, plant hormones not only help prevent menopausal symptoms; they may protect you from breast cancer. Breast cancer rates are dramatically lower in Japan than in the United States. There may be other factors involved, however, such as childbearing habits and low-fat diets. After menopause, high-fat diets can increase your risk of heart attack and stroke — no matter how much estrogen you take. Meanwhile, bad habits such as heavy intake of coffee and alcohol and smoking can increase your risk of osteoporosis. Right now, most doctors will tell you to go ahead and add as much soy as you want to your diet. It may well help; and it certainly can't hurt!

Phytoestrogens can be taken orally or even in creams, which can be applied to your body. Creams are quasi-natural, however, because the plant hormones they contain are modified in a lab. Because plant-based hormones contain chemicals that are similar but not identical to your natural estrogen, questions remain about their use.

49. Know Where to Find Phytoestrogens

Here's a list of phytoestrogens you can purchase at health food stores. Again, these may help with a myriad of menopausal discomforts and may possibly protect you from heart disease:

- Agave *(Agave americana)*. One dose is ¼–1 teaspoon or 1–5 ml of juice of the leaves.
- Alfalfa *(Medicago sativa)*
- Amerikanerischer schneeball or schneeball
- Black cohosh *(Cimicifuga racemosa)*
- Black currant
- Black haw *(Viburnum prunifolium)* or Viorne obier *(V. opulis)*
- Bockshornklee
- Casses *(Ribes nigrum)*
- Chaste tree *(Vitex agnus castus)*
- Cramp bark or guelder rose
- Dandelion *(Taraxacum officinale)*
- Devil's club *(Chamalirium luteum)*
- Dong Quai/Dang Gui *(Angelica sinensis)*
- Fenugreek *(Trigonella foenumgraecum)*. Good for hot flashes.
- Garden sage *(Salvia officinalis)*. Good for night sweats.
- Gemeines Kreuzkraut
- Ginseng *(Panax ginseng)*
- Groundsel *(Senecio vulgaris)*

- Hop *(Humulus lupulus)*
- Hopfen
- Licorice *(Glycyrrhiza glabra).* Note: this can be toxic in high doses, causing high blood pressure and water retention.
- Liferoot *(Senecio aureus)*
- Lowenzahn
- Motherwort *(Leonurus cardiaca).* Good for night sweats.
- Nettle *(Urtica dioica* or *U. Urens)*
- Peony *(Paeonia officinalis).* Frequently combined with Dong Quai/Dang Gui.
- Pomegranate *(Punica granatum).* These seeds pack 1.7 grams of estrone for every 3 ounces, just eat the seeds instead of spitting them out when you consume the fruit; or make them into a smoothie in the blender, or grind them and infuse in oil to make your own estrogen cream.
- Red clover *(Trifolium pratense)*
- Rose family (raspberry, strawberry, sweetbrier, hawthorn, dog rose, hagrose, eglantier). Rose hips are an excellent source of flavonoids.
- Sarsaparilla *(Smilax officinalis* or *S. regelii).* Jamaican is considered best, with Mexican and Honduran following closely.
- Saw palmetto *(Serenoa repens)*
- Schlangenwurzel
- Schwarze or Schwarze Johannisbeere

- Wild yam (*Dioscorea villosa* and all five hundred related species). Progesterone cream derived from wild yam has been shown to reverse osteoporosis.
- Yarrow (*Achillea millefolium*)

50. Take This Book to Your Health Care Provider

Protecting yourself from heart disease encompasses a range of decisions, and some of them are very difficult ones to make. For starters, it's not easy to weigh the risks of heart disease against the risks of hormone replacement therapy, especially if you're concerned about breast cancer. But if you're past menopause, a discussion about heart disease and hormone replacement therapy necessarily entails another discussion about your risk of breast cancer. That's because the incidence of breast cancer in Western nations dramatically rises after menopause, and some studies show that HRT contributes to this increase. (Note: If you're on HRT and are diagnosed with breast cancer, doctors will simply take you off hormone replacement therapy, which completely eliminates the problem and restores your survival rate to that of the general population. Many medical papers also suggest that women undergoing breast cancer treatment can still be on HRT. It is not necessarily a conflict.)

For the record, heart disease kills more women than breast cancer, and HRT can definitely lower your cholesterol levels, lower your risk of getting heart disease, and reduce your risk of dying from heart disease. Furthermore, if you are at greater risk for osteoporosis (we're all at risk, but women who exercise or have heavier bones will not develop it as quickly), HRT stops bone loss. In fact, if started in the first few years after menopause, HRT will even increase bone mass. Remember: Hip and spinal fractures can be very debilitating (often life threatening) and can truly affect quality of life.

You will also want to discuss with your health care provider the advantages of conventional HRT over natural hormone replacement therapy and balance all those factors with other chronic health problems you may have. Then there are, of course, all of the lifestyle modifications raised earlier to consider, such as quitting smoking, diet, and exercise.

As you sort through the pages of this little book, you'll find it's packed with a lot of information mined from many sources. You have in your hands a powerful shield against heart disease: correct information. And it is information many doctors don't know because much of what was taught in medical school until very recently was what we knew about heart disease predominantly in white males. Learn this information and pass it on to both older family members (your mother and grandmother or aunts and great-aunts) as well as younger relatives (your daughters, nieces, and grandnieces, especially if they smoke). By quitting smoking (numbers 1 through 10), adjusting your diet (numbers 11 through 20), exercising (numbers 21 through 30), lowering blood pressure and cholesterol (numbers 31 through 39), protecting yourself from the sexually transmitted disease chlamydia (number 40), and making an informed choice about either natural hormone therapy or conventional HRT, you can dramatically lower your risk of heart disease. I hope you will take all this good information to heart!

Glossary

Note: This list is not exhaustive. It's more of a reminder list based on some of the key points I'd like you to remember from this book.

Aerobic activity: any activity that causes the heart to pump harder and faster, causing you to breathe faster, which increases the level of oxygen in the bloodstream.

Anorexia nervosa: "a loss of appetite due to mental disorder." People with anorexia refuse to eat any food at all, starving themselves.

Antihypertensive drug: a drug designed to lower blood pressure, sometimes called a blood thinner.

Antioxidants: vitamins A, C, E, and beta-carotene, found in colored (nongreen) fruits and vegetables. Antioxidants prevent the oxidation of cell membranes, which can lead to cancer; they are the "cancer-fighting soldiers."

Binge-eating disorder: refers to compulsive overeating, or bingeing without purging.

Bulimia nervosa: bingeing followed by purging in the form of self-induced vomiting, laxative/diuretic abuse, or abusing other medications to induce weight loss.

Carbohydrates: the building blocks of most foods, which provide energy to the body to fuel the central nervous system; they help the body use vitamins, minerals, amino acids, and other nutrients.

Cholesterol: a whitish, waxy fat made in vast quantities by the liver. (*See also* HDL; LDL)

Complex carbohydrates: sophisticated carbohydrate foods that have larger molecules in them, such as grain foods and foods high in fiber.

Endometrium: the lining of the uterus, which shelters a fertilized egg and secretes embryo-nourishing substances. This is what sheds during menstruation.

Fatty acids: crucial nutrients for cells, which also regulate hormone production.

Fiber: part of a plant that cannot be digested, which can lower cholesterol levels or improve regularity; also causes a slower rise in glucose levels, which lowers the body's insulin requirements.

Follicle stimulating hormone (FSH): released by the pituitary gland, this hormone stimulates the growth of the follicles containing the eggs, which, as they grow, produce the hormone estrogen.

HDL: high-density lipoproteins, known as the "good" cholesterol.

Hydrogenation: process that converts liquid fat to semisolid fat by adding hydrogen.

Hypertension (high blood pressure): high tension or force exerted on the artery walls; a condition that damages the small blood vessels as well as the larger arteries.

Hysterectomy: surgical removal of the uterus.

LDL: low-density lipoproteins, known as the "bad" cholesterol.

Lean body mass: body tissue that is not fat.

Menarche: the first menstrual period.

Modifiable risk factor: a risk factor that can be changed by alterations in lifestyle or diet.

Obesity: when a person weighs more than 20 percent of her ideal weight for her age and height.

Omega-3 fatty acids: naturally present in fish that swim in cold waters; crucial for brain tissue; are all poly-unsaturated, and not only lower cholesterol levels but are said to protect against heart disease.

Orlistat: an antiobesity drug that blocks the absorption of almost one-third of the fat one consumes.

Osteoporosis: literally means "porous bones." A condition common to postmenopausal women.

Phytoestrogens: plant estrogens said to be therapeutically beneficial for symptoms of menopause.

Pituitary gland: also called the master gland, the pituitary gland keeps track of your age, begins your reproductive cycle at puberty, controls your body during pregnancy, and ends your cycle at menopause.

Progesterone: often referred to as the pregnancy hormone, this is the hormone responsible for preparing the lining of the uterus for pregnancy.

Progestin: synthetic progesterone.

Prophylactic: preventive.

Risk marker: a risk factor that cannot be changed, such as age or genes.

Saturated fat: a fat solid at room temperature (from animal sources) that stimulates the body to produce LDL, or "bad" cholesterol.

Soluble fiber: fiber that is water soluble, or dissolves in water; forms a gel in the body that traps fats and lowers cholesterol.

Stroke: occurs when a blood clot travels to the brain and stops the flow of blood and oxygen carried to the nerve cells in that area, at which point cells may die or vital body functions controlled by the brain may be temporarily or permanently damaged.

Systolic pressure: one of the readings in a blood pressure measurement; the pressure occurring during the heart's contraction.

Trans-fatty acids (hydrogenated oils): harmful, man-made fats that not only raise the level of "bad" cholesterol (LDL) in the bloodstream, but lower the amount of "good" cholesterol (HDL) that's already there; produced through the process of hydrogenation.

Triglycerides: a combination of saturated, monounsaturated, and polyunsaturated fatty acids and glycerol.

Type 2 diabetes: non-insulin-dependent diabetes mellitus (NIDDM), also called late-onset or mature-onset diabetes because it's usually diagnosed after age forty-five; the body is either not producing enough insulin or the insulin it does produce cannot be used efficiently.

Unsaturated fat: known as "good fat" because it doesn't cause the body to produce "bad" cholesterol, and it increases the levels of "good" cholesterol; partially solid or liquid at room temperature.

Urethra: a tube that connects the bladder to the outside of the body.

Uterus: more of a vessel or receptacle for the fetus than an organ; controlled entirely by hormones.

Bibliography

"A Complex Question of Odds: Hormones versus No Treatment." *Health Facts* 18 (January 1993).

"Anger with an 'A' Spells Trouble." *Countdown USA: Countdown to a Healthy Heart*, Allegheny General Hospital and Voluntary Hospitals of America, Inc. (1990).

Apple, Rima D. (ed.). *Women, Health and Medicine in America: A Historical Handbook*. Piscataway, N.J.: Rutgers University Press, 1992.

Arsenault, Gillian, M.D. *Breast Cancer Epidemiology*. Unpublished report, 1996.

Beard, M.D., Mary K., and Lindsay R. Curtis, M.D. *Menopause and the Years Ahead*. Tuscon, Ariz.: Fisher Books, 1988.

Bequaert Holmes, Helen. "A Call to Heal Medicine." *Feminist Perspectives in Medical Ethics*. Helen Bequaert Holmes and Laura M. Purdy (eds.). Bloomington, Ind.: Indiana University Press, 1992.

Berndl, Leslie, R.D., M.Sc. "Understanding Fat." *Diabetes Dialogue* 42, no. 1 (Spring 1995).

Beyers, Joanne, R.D. "How Sweet It Is!" *Diabetes Dialogue* 42, no. 1 (Spring 1995).

Biermann, June, and Barbara Toohey. *The Diabetic's Book.* New York: Perigee Books, 1992.

The Boston Women's Health Book Collective. *The New Our Bodies, Ourselves.* New York: Simon & Schuster, 1992.

Brewster, Wendy. "New study challenges cancer, estrogen link." *Reuters Health Summary* (March 29, 1997).

British Columbia Women's Community Consultation Report. *The Challenges Ahead for Women's Health.* B.C. Women's Hospital and Health Centre Society, Vancouver (1995).

Brody, Jane E. "Personal Health." *New York Times* (April 2, 1997).

Canadian Diabetes Association "You Are What You Eat." *Equilibrium,* no. 1 (1996).

Canadian Hypertension Society. "High Blood Pressure and Drug Treatment." (1999).

"Carbohydrate Counting: A New Way to Plan Meals." American Diabetes Association. January 1999. http://www.diabetes.com.

Casper, Robert F., and Alcide Chapdelaine. "Estrogen and Interrupted Progestin: A New Concept for Menopausal Hormone Replacement Therapy." *American Journal of Obstetrics and Gynecology* 168 (April 1993).

Chaddock, Brenda, C.D.E. "Foul Weather Fitness: The Hardest Part Is Getting Started." *Canadian Pharmacy Journal* (March 1996).

———. "The Magic of Exercise." *Canadian Pharmacy Journal* (September 1995).

"Cholesterol and Women." *Health News,* from the publishers of the *New England Journal of Medicine* (November 21, 1995).

Cicala, Roger S., M.D. *The Heart Disease Sourcebook.* Los Angeles: Lowell House, 1998.

Clarke, Bill. "Action Figures." *Diabetes Dialogue* 43, no. 3 (Fall 1996).

"Combat Job Stress: Does Work Make You Sick?" http://www.convoke.com/markjr/ cjstress.html (12 February 1999).

Coney, Sandra. *The Menopause Industry: How the Medical Establishment Exploits Women.* San Francisco: Hunter House, 1994.

Costin, Carolyn. *The Eating Disorder Sourcebook.* Los Angeles: Lowell House, 1999.

Cronier, Claire, M.Sc., R.D. "Sweetest Choices." *Diabetes Dialogue* 44, no. 1 (Spring 1997).

Delaney, Kathy, R.N., B.S.N., and Marie R. Squillace. *Living with Heart Disease.* Los Angeles: Lowell House, 1998.

DeMarco, Carolyn. "Keys to the Highway." *Wellness MD* 3, no. 6 (November/December 1993).

———. *Take Charge of Your Body: A Woman's Guide to Health.* Winlaw, B.C.: The Last Laugh, 1990.

Dickens, B. M. "The Doctrine of Informed Consent." In *Justice Beyond Orwell.* R. S. Abella and M. L. Rothman (eds.). Montreal: Yvon Blais, 1985: 243–63.

"Diet and Breast Cancer." *Nutrition Research Newsletter* 13 (September 1994): 101. Adapted from *Archives of*

Internal Medicine (August 22, 1994) and *British Journal of Cancer* (September 1994).

Doepel, Laurie, K. "Looking at Menopause's Role in Osteoporosis." *Journal of the American Medical Association* 254, no. 17 (November 1, 1985).

Doress, Paula Brown, Diana Laskin Seigal, and the Midlife and Older Women Book Project in Cooperation with the Boston Women's Health Collective. *Ourselves Growing Older.* New York: Simon & Schuster, 1987.

Dori, Stehlin, "A Little Lite Reading." http://www.fda.gov/fdac/foodlabel/diabetes.html (11 January 1999).

Dreher, Henry, and Alice D. Domar, Ph.D. *Healing Mind, Healthy Woman.* New York: Holt, 1996.

Engel, June V., Ph. D., "Beyond Vitamins: Phytochemicals to Help Fight Disease." *Health News* 14 (June 1996).

———. "Eating Fibre." *Diabetes Dialogue* 44, no.1 (Spring 1997).

"Estrogen Replacement Therapy and Breast Cancer Risk," *Cancer Researcher Weekly* (May 10, 1993).

"Estrogens in Vegetables May Reduce Hot Flashes and Breast Cancer Risk, Cornell University Nutritionist Says." Cornell University press release (February 17, 1994).

Etchells, E., et al. "Disclosure." *Canadian Medical Association Journal* 155 (1996): 387–91.

———. "Voluntariness." *Canadian Medical Association Journal* 155 (1996): 1083–86.

Etchells, E., and Gilbert Sharpe, et al. "Consent." *Canadian Medical Association Journal* 155 (1006): 177–80.

"Evidence for Estrogen." *The Medical Post* (April 9, 1996): 75–76.

"Exercise: Guidelines to a Healthier You." Patient information. Bayer, Inc. Healthcare Division, distributed 1997.

Farquhar, Andrew, M.D. "Exercising Essentials." *Diabetes Dialogue* 43, no. 3 (Fall 1996): 6–8.

Findlay, Deborah, and Leslia Miller. "Medical Power and Women's Bodies." In *Women, Medicine and Health*. B. S. Bolaria and R. Bolaria (eds.). Halifax, NS: Fernwood, 1994.

Finucane, Fanchon F., "Decreased Risk of Stroke Among Postmenopausal Hormone Users: Results from a National Cohort" *Journal of the American Medical Association* 269 (June 2, 1993).

"Following the Patient With Chronic Disease." *Patient Care Canada* 7, no. 5 (May 1996): 22–38.

"Food Alone Can't Always Provide Requisite Nutrition." *Globe and Mail* (September 28, 1998).

Food and Drug Administration. "Nutrient Claims Guide for Individual Foods." Special Report, Focus on Food Labeling. FDA Publication no. 95-2289.

"Food and Exercise: Guidelines to a Healthier You." Patient information. Bayer, Inc. Healthcare Division, distributed 1997.

Fugh-Berman, Adriane, *Alternative Medicine: What Works*. Tucson, Ariz.: Odonian Press, 1996.

"Getting to the Roots of a Vegetarian Diet." Baltimore, Md.: Vegetarian Resource Group, 1997.

Greenberg, Brigitte. "Stress Hormone Linked to High-Fat Snacking in Women." *Associated Press* (April 4, 1998).

Harrison, Pam. "Rethinking Obesity." *Family Practice* (March 11, 1996).

Healy, Barnadine, M.D. *A New Prescription for Women's Health: Getting the Best Medical Care in a Man's World.* New York: Penguin Books, 1995.

"The Heart Healthy Kitchen." *Countdown USA: Countdown to a Healthy Heart.* Allegheny General Hospital and Voluntary Hospitals of America, Inc., 1990.

Heimlic, Jane. *What Your Doctor Won't Tell You: The Complete Guide to the Latest in Alternative Medicine.* New York: Harper-Perennial, 1990.

Hendler, Saul Sheldon, M.D., Ph.D. *The Doctors' Vitamin and Mineral Encyclopedia.* New York: Fireside Books, 1990.

Henkel, Gretchen. *Making the Estrogen Decision.* Los Angeles: Lowell House, 1997.

"High Blood Pressure and Drug Treatment." Patient information leaflet published by the Canadian Hypertension Society.

"High Levels of Saturated Fat Found to Promote Ovarian Cancer." *New York Times.* (September 21, 1994, sec. C, p. 10).

Ho, Marian, M.Sc., R.D. "Learning Your ABCs, Part Two." *Diabetes Dialogue* 43, no. 3 (Fall 1996).

"Hostility and Heart Risk." *Reuters Health Summary* (April 22, 1997).

"How to Deal With Stress." http://www.backrelief.com/stress (12 February 1999).

Hufnagel, Vicki, M.D. *No More Hysterectomies.* New York: New American Library, 1989.

Hunter, J. E. and T. H. Applewhite. "Reassessment of Trans Fatty Acid Availability in the U.S. Diet." *American Journal of Clinical Nutrition* 54 (1991): 363–69.

Hurley, Jane, and Stephen Schmidt. "Going with the Grain." *Nutrition Action* (October 1994): 10–11.

"Hysterectomy and a Woman's Sex Life." *Women's Letter* (January 1991).

"IFIC Review: Intense Sweeteners: Effects on Appetite and Weight Management." International Food Information Council, 1100 Connecticut Avenue N.W., Suite 430, Washington DC 20036 (November 1995).

"IFIC Review: Uses and Nutritional Impact of Fat Reduction Ingredients." International Food Information Council, 1100 Connecticut Avenue N.W., Suite 430, Washington DC 20036 (October 1995).

Jovanovic-Peterson, Lois, M.D., June Biermann, and Barbara Toohey. *The Diabetic Woman: All Your Questions Answered.* New York: G. P. Putnam's Sons, 1996.

"Kicking the Habit: At Last, a Treatment That Combats Craving." http://www.sciam.com (*Scientific American*) (2 January 2000).

Kuczmarski, R. J., K. M. Flegal, S. M. Campbell, and C. L. Johnson. "Increasing Prevalence of Overweight Among U.S. Adults: The National Health and Nutrition Examination Surveys, 1960 to 1991." *Journal of the American Medical Association* 272 (1994): 205–11.

Lark, Susan M., M.D. *The Menopause Self-Help Book.* Berkeley, Calif.: Celestial Arts, 1990.

Lee, John R., M.D. *What Your Doctor May Not Tell You About Menopause.* New York: Warner Books, 1996.

Lemonick, Michael D. "Eat Your Heart Out." *Time* (July 19, 1999).

Leutwyler, Kristin. "Dying to Be Thin." *Women's Health* 9, no. 2 (Summer 1998).

Levine, R. J. *Ethics and Regulation of Clinical Research.* New Haven, Conn.: Yale University Press, 1988.

Lindsay, Robert. "Prevention and Treatment of Osteoporosis." *Lancet* 341, (March 27, 1993).

Linton, Marilyn. *Taking Charge by Taking Care.* Toronto: Macmillan Canada, 1996.

Mastroianni, Anna C., Ruth Faden, and Daniel Federman (eds.). *Women and Health Research: Ethical and Legal Issues of Including Women in Clinical Studies,* vol. 1. Washington, DC: National Academy Press, 1994.

Morrison, Judith H. *The Book of Ayurveda.* New York: Simon & Schuster, 1995.

Muhlestein, Joseph, B., et al. "Increased Incidence of Chlamydia Species Within the Coronary Arteries of Patients with Symptomatic Atherosclerotic versus Other Forms of Cardiovascular Disease." *Journal of the Ameican College of Cardiology* 27 (1996): 1555–61.

Nechas, Eileen, and Denise Foley. *Unequal Treatment: What You Don't Know About How Women Are Mistreated by the Medical Community.* New York: Simon and Schuster, 1994.

"New Study Challenges Cancer, Estrogen Link." *Times Colonist* (March 29, 1997).

"Olestra: Yes or No?" Excerpted from *University of California at Berkeley Wellness Letter,* c. Health Associates, 1996 in *Diabetes Dialogue* 43, no. 3 (Fall 1996).

Ontario Task Force on the Primary Prevention of Cancer. *Recommendations for the Primary Prevention of Cancer: Report of the Ontario Task Force on the Primary Prevention of Cancer.* Toronto, March 1995. Presented to the Ontario Ministry of Health.

Orbach, Susie. *Fat Is a Feminist Issue.* New York: Berkeley Books, 1990.

Osteoporosis Society of Canada. "Menopause: Let's Talk About It." Booklet, 1996.

Patient Information. The National Digestive Diseases Information Clearinghouse, (NDDIC), a service of the National Institute of Diabetes and Digestive and Kidney Diseases, part of the National Institutes of Health, under the U.S. Public Health Service. 1996, National Digestive Diseases Information Clearinghouse, licensed to Medical Strategies, Inc.

Pearson, Cynthia. "FDA Waffles on Premarin Decision." *Network News* 15 (July/August 1990).

Perry, Susan, and Katherine O'Hanlan, M.D. *Natural Menopause: The Complete Guide to a Woman's Most Misunderstood Passage.* New York: Addison-Wesley Publishing, 1992.

"Pocket Partner: A Guide to Healthy Food Choices." Booklet. Canadian Diabetes Association, distributed 1997.

"Postmenopausal Osteoporosis and Preventative Measures." *American Family Physician* 45, no. 3 (March 1992).

"Prevention and Treatment of Obesity: Application to Type 2 Diabetes (Technical Review)." *Diabetes Care* 20: 1744–66 (1997).

"Putting Fun Back into Food." International Food Information Council, 1100 Connecticut Avenue N.W., Suite 430, Washington DC 20036 (1997).

"Q&A about Fatty Acids and Dietary Fats." International Food Information Council, 1100 Connecticut Avenue N.W., Suite 430, Washington DC 20036 (1997).

Randall, Lee. "Is HRT for Me?" *Weight Watchers* 26 (February 1993).

"Replacement Therapy for Reducing Cardiovascular Disease." *Western Journal of Medicine* (May 1993).

Rosenthal, M. Sara. *The Breast Sourcebook*, 2d ed. Los Angeles: Lowell House, 1999.

———. *The Gynecological Sourcebook*, 3d ed. Los Angeles: Lowell House, 1999.

———. *Managing Diabetes for Women*. Toronto: Macmillan Canada, 1999.

———. *Managing Your Diabetes*. Toronto: Macmillan Canada, 1998.

Rosser, Sue V. *Women's Health—Missing from U.S. Medicine.* Bloomington, Ind.: Indiana University Press, 1994.

Seto, Carol, R.D., C.D.E. "Nutrition Labeling—U.S. Style." *Diabetes Dialogue* 42, no.1 (Spring 1995).

Sherwin, Susan. "Feminist and Medical Ethics: Two Different Approaches to Contextual Ethics." In

Feminist Perspectives in Medical Ethics. Helen Bequaert Holmes and Laura M. Purdy (eds.). Bloomington, Ind.: Indiana University Press, 1992.

———. *Patient No Longer: Feminist Ethics and Health Care.* Philadelphia: Temple University Press, 1984.

Shimer, Porter. *Keeping Fitness Simple: 500 Tips for Fitting Exercise into Your Life.* Pownal, Vt.: Storey Books, 1998.

Siegfried J. Kra, M.D., F.A.C.P. *What Every Woman Must Know About Heart Disease.* New York: Warner Books, 1996.

"Sorting Out the Facts About Fat." International Food Information Council, 1100 Connecticut Avenue N.W., Suite 430, Washington DC 20036 (1997).

Steinberg, W. M. "Menopause and Breast Cancer." *Patient Care* (May 1993):8.

"10 Tips to Healthy Eating." American Dietetic Association and National Center for Nutrition and Dietetics (NCND) (April 1994).

Warren, Virgina, L. "Feminist Directions in Medical Ethics." In *Feminist Perspectives in Medical Ethics.* Helen Bequaert Holmes and Laura M. Purdy (eds.). Bloomington, Ind.: Indiana University Press, 1992.

Weed, Susun S. *Menopausal Years: The Wise Woman Way— Alternative Approaches for Women 30–90.* Woodstock, N.Y.: Ash Tree Publishing, 1992.

Whiteford, Linda. "Political Economy, Gender and the Social Production of Health and Illness." In *Gender and Health.* C. Sargent and C. Brettell (eds.). Toronto: Prentice-Hall, 1996.

Willett, W. C., et al. "Intake of Trans Fatty Acids and Risk of Coronary Heart Disease Among Women." *Lancet* 341 (1993): 581–85.

"Women Find Themselves Courted by Pharmaceutical Firms." *Associated Press* (July 20, 1998).

Wright, Jonathan V., and John Morgenthaler. *Natural Hormone Replacement.* Petaluma, Calif.: Smart Publications, 1997.

"Your Medical Test Guide." *Health for Women* VIII, no. 2 (Spring/Summer 1998).

Zimmerman, Mary K. "The Women's Health Movement: A Critique of Medical Enterprise and the Position of Women." In *Analysing Gender.* M. Farle and B. Hess (eds.). Thousand Oaks, Calif.: Sage, 1987.

Index